Think and Grow Fit

◆

A Rational Person's Guide to Getting Fit and Staying That Way Forever

Mark Clemens

iUniverse, Inc.
New York   Bloomington

iUniverse books may be ordered through booksellers or by contacting:

iUniverse
1663 Liberty Drive
Bloomington, IN 47403
www.iuniverse.com
1-800-Authors (1-800-288-4677)

Because of the dynamic nature of the Internet, any Web addresses or links
contained in this book may have changed since publication and may no
longer be valid. The views expressed in this work are solely those of the
author and do not necessarily reflect the views of the publisher, and the
publisher hereby disclaims any responsibility for them.

ISBN: 978-1-4401-9266-1 (sc)
ISBN: 978-1-4401-9267-8 (ebook)

Printed in the United States of America

iUniverse rev. date: 12/23/2009

Contents

1

A New Age; A New You

Friends, what if a new training program really worked? Might you not then go from Jo or Joanne Average to Olympic Starlet Dara Torres or Grandfather of Fitness Jack LaLanne? If you did, who would like you anymore? Surely not all of your friends who love all of that "soda, pretzels, and beer," to paraphrase the mellow Nat King Cole song of the 1960s. These are all part of the American good life of ease, which we're all supposed to seek out and enjoy as if it's our birthright. Turning into an over-forty athlete just might turn you into a tofu-craving marathoner hooked on green tea and multivitamins. That would make you into a real freak of nature—a truly certifiable Health Nut as they always call it. No one could ever like anyone this odd, could they?

Of course, most people say that none of that "athletic stuff" ever works for them. Maybe they've tried their hand at it and failed not just once, but numerous times. Maybe they've tried every new diet from the Mayo Clinic diet of the 1970s to the Atkins diet of the 1990s, only to have every pound come right back on. Maybe they've bought and garage-saled off an exercycle and/or a Bowflex gym set. Maybe they've even tried (yet again) the latest fat burner, only to find that they got no more from it than a severe case of the jitters. So what's the use? You might as well give up, right? Maybe, but it's likely that you won't.

All I can hope is that this time will be the one that really makes the difference. That's what this book is all about. So I'm asking you to take on the role of Health Nut for a while. It won't be easy, as you'll have to give up a lot of people in the "Normal Majority": friends, relatives, neighbors, and maybe even a few TV icons who, you are sure, would never stoop to a salad a day, popping twenty to thirty supplements, or swimming a mile instead of eating French-dipped beef sandwiches with the gang on their lunch hour.

But you know that your Not Okay Health Nut behavior will work eventually. The only real trick is keeping at it, right? Maybe it's even doing it without anyone becoming the wiser. The bottom line, though, is that you know it's right and it's what you must do—just like brushing your teeth—if you really want to win. How can you disagree?

Yet agreeing with me just might also mean following the lead of a guy who wears jumpsuits (the peerless, now ninety-five-year-old Jack LaLanne) or a woman who looks like a movie star, "middle-aged" Olympic winner Dara Torres, or even a real star (though some think they aren't real people) such as Jane Fonda. How could all of that ever be doable for feet-on-the-ground, realistic and sensible you? Come along and dream with me a little.

I always wanted to be like Jack LaLanne, the guy on TV my mother idolized in the early 1960s. Also, I didn't want to be fat on my first day of high school. I was obese—yes, really flabby—back then, you see. Couldn't ever get a girlfriend with all that fat, right? Okay, some say it's your personality that counts, but do you trust them? I didn't then and I don't now.

Anyway, that's why there are so many examples of looking good and getting beach ready throughout the body of what follows. Being a high school kid after a girlfriend, looking good in the mirror, getting ready for the beach, and the like not only made more sense to me but seemed so much more effective over the long haul than the old doctor's scare tactics like: "If you don't lose the pounds by Christmas, you won't live to see the tree" threats. No one has ever kept it off after losing it like that, have they?

It takes a lot of GOFHW (good old-fashioned hard work)—dedication, that is—to go from average to special. It takes even more to stay there and go beyond, even when you're gung ho and maybe encouraged by a favorite hero or a very good personal trainer.

But how can you ever get into it like that? How can you keep from saying, "What's the use?" Why bother in the first place? What's more important right now that I should really be doing? Besides, the Normal Majority, the people who ask these dreary questions, think that being average is okay, good enough for anyone and in fact better than things are the world over, Third World countries in particular. And they're right, right?

Personally, I never got along well with the Normal Majority—the big people with all of the answers. So I suppose I am a born Health Nut (though I believe that thinking of myself as a health-conscious person is whole lot better). Yet, when I think about it, I feel lucky in spite of all their criticism and rejection. I always knew that these Normal People had their own agendas when they tried to convince me they were only thinking of me. Further, none of them really looked like Jack LaLanne or Bob Hoffman (then active US Olympic coach) or, later on, Jane Fonda. They all looked pretty unshapely, not even close to how I wanted to be. So how could I possibly take them seriously, especially when it came to fitness?

That being said, I knew I was pretty much on my own, maybe like you are, knowing little more than that I wanted to look good for a cute girl. That made me cut my diet to 1,000 calories a day to lose the weight. But going from a forty-inch waist to a twenty-eight-inch one was not going to be the be all end and end all; I knew that. Keeping it off was going to be a battle in itself, and getting really athletic: "You've got to be a football hero to get along with the beautiful girls," if you remember the song, was going to be an even worse ordeal.

Becoming an athlete took years of experimentation and periods of discouragement. And I felt like a crook doing the good things that I did. The Normal Majority high school coaches and teachers back then didn't approve of what I was good at: weightlifting. It makes you muscle-bound and vain, they said. Besides, you can't get a letter in it. Then too, my mother didn't approve of vitamins, so I ended up sneaking them into my bedroom. (That's a little like Jane Fonda, whom Nixon busted for smuggling. Her contraband turned out to be vitamins.)

But in spite of the hassles, I was determined to be a champion, just like Rocky Balboa in *Rocky I,* about whom you'll hear a lot later on. That's why in 1978, twelve years after I graduated from high school, I finally won my weight class in the state power-lifting tournament. I'm still into being megahealthy because it feels and looks good (and it makes people think I'm younger). Can you relate to *any* of this? I hope so.

Today, when America seems to be suffering from an obesity epidemic—the primary cause of the other maladies that depress our great country—what this book is all about just may be timely. You see, I think we all need to start focusing on low-fat and low-carb eating, supplementing wisely, and never missing a workout. That's a whole lot different from being into dollar burgers or the R&R (rest and relaxation) of the good life, with its Thanksgiving and Fourth of July pig-outs, to say nothing of the endless hazy, crazy days of summer with their sodas and pretzels and beer.

It's also a lot different than idolizing that two-hundred-fifty-pound halfback, the heavyweight boxing champion, or the seven-foot basketball star, none of whom ever amount to much after they're too old (according to the Normal Majority) to play. Rather, it's about replacing them all with your neighborhood fifty-year-old marathoners and triathletes, or maybe a forty-two-year-old Dara Torres who is looking forward to another Olympian gold medal when she hits forty-six. Then it's about making sure that your kids do the same.

This book asks this serious question: how can there still be two classes of people in this great country, the Normal Majority and the "Health Nuts"—the folks who think they just might be able to look forty-two when going on sixty-two? Could that be you? If we have a health problem in this country—and we do unless you think the diabetes, heart, and cholesterol numbers aren't all that bad in relation to the AIDS problem in Africa—why are we still listening to the advice of the people who make it all worse?

This book asks how, though they are considered to be so sensible or mature, the less healthy Normal Majority can still be taken seriously. In other words, how can the Health Nuts be in a minority position when what they have to say and the way they live are such important models during this time of increasing flab, diabetes, and heart trouble right here on every Main Street in our country. And most importantly, why are these people looking up to the Normal Majority?

I can't just be rhetorical about this, right? I have to have a theory. So ... here goes: my guess is that Health Nuts are perceived by the Normal Majority, the folks in power, as unrealistic or ephemeral, as people who do not act their ages. Of course, the Health Nuts think that their Normal Majority critics are right; therefore, they too are part of the problem. This causes a very unhealthy atmosphere for the person who's trying to make it. He has to do so in spite of feeling inferior, even a little crazy, in fact. Maybe that will change sometime soon, just as women's liberation eventually made it unthinkable to use the word "girl" instead of "woman"—but we aren't there yet.

One of the cardinal sins in our country, something that is wholly unforgivable, is to act younger than your age. You can be forgiven for acting older, but acting younger is cause for severe criticism, such as "What are you trying to prove? You're not a spring chicken anymore" and the like. The presumed rationale is that doing so is phony. In other words, you're a fraud as a human. The real person, so the Normal Majority thinks, should be slowing down, losing a zest for living, becoming out of shape and expecting to step back from intense living (whether one wants to retire or not). That is their only appropriate game plan for you as you to continue to age and die at eighty (even though some who study longevity, with good reason, are shooting for 140).

Being a Health Nut, according to them, is what you should have gotten out of your system back in high school. This generally means that running a number of times around the block (let's say doing a five-mile run before going to work), saying no to Christmas cookies, refusing invitations to TGIF or Thanksgiving pig-outs, to say nothing of daily trips to the golden arches for lunch, are absurdities that only high school kids out for the team should be into. The same goes for buying all those pesky pills from the vitamin shop, which you shouldn't have needed anyway because you're eating those three square meals a day from the four food groups.

In a day and age of supplement stores, health clubs, nutritional sophistication, and people like Dara Torres, Jane Fonda, and Jack LaLanne—who have not only stayed active and fit but have actually gotten better with time—I think it's time to take a closer look at what we are all *supposed* to think of as the American good life. Might not this image, based on the Normal Majority's expectations of how you're supposed to look and live at specific ages, need some changing right now? Might it not be that the Health Nuttiness of eating right, supplementing wisely, and working out should be seen as more appropriate and better for everyone than the three grocery-store square meals from the four food groups, a "little bit of walking now and then," and the annual checkup with the MD (unless you're going there before your appointment to see if the latest new wonder drug is right for you).

The Health Nut stigma may be the primary reason so many come back to the Normal Majority side after trying to get into a healthy lifestyle. They just can't stay at dieting, supplementing, and working out, knowing that this puts them into the category of Health Nut. These are things you really need to do if you want to look good as the years go on. But doing them "just ain't cool" in most social circles (and no one can stand derogatory comments from their betters). That's the prevalent opinion of the Normal Majority and, sadly, even of those who dare to try their hand at being a Health Nut. Friends, with associates like these and an attitude like that, you haven't got a prayer.

Of course, time and money are also considerations. With long commutes, family obligations, and just so many hours in the day, time to work out can seem nonexistent. And money is tight in this economy. Where are the extra dollars for the health club memberships, the organic food from the co-op, and the bottles of supplements? Tons of other books have answers to these questions. We all know that people will make time for what's important and find money for what they care about. We *do* all *know* that, don't we? We all know that the means to do anything follows from the desire to do it in the first place. Where there's a will, there's a way.

The Normal Majority believes that you cannot turn back the clock. That's another huge part of the issue. Two things are for sure: death and taxes. This translates into: you're going to get dumpy, and there are no two ways about it. "Take it from me," they love to remind you—even when they are chronologically your junior. "I'm more seasoned and wiser than you are." Therefore, it's fitting that you go with the flow and age gracefully.

Despite anti-aging remedies that include diet, energy, skin care and exercise articles all over the Internet, the Normal Majority believes that using them is only doing cosmetic work on yourself—despite the fact that these methods actually make cellular changes. Serious folks, especially adults over forty, are expected to be involved only in their careers, making things right for their children, and being responsible in the community—falling asleep at PTA or church council meetings. They're also supposed to be in love with AARP.

If you have thoughts like these going on in your head, it will sooner than later become impossible to stick with the best of your intentions. Just hit a tough period during one of your workouts and you'll see what I mean. Such thoughts just may make you leave the gym early, which I think of as a cardinal sin. This happens all too often, and that's why New Year's resolutions never work, even though you know they should.

Friends, you have got to get away from this Normal Majority–type thinking. Give it up for good. It is what is causing your trouble, and that's true whether you're forty-two or sixty-two. If you don't, you will be forever starting out on January 2 only to be back to square one by March 1.

This will all be much easier with a spouse who's on your side—if not right there *at* your side—when you're on the stationary bike or treadmill. So sharpen up those negotiation skills. You need him or her to be there for you. The same goes for having some new health-conscious friends, even if they, too, are still silly enough to call themselves Health Nuts. You can all work on refusing to put yourselves down as soon as you get to know each other better.

Just forget the quick-fix mania. It's going to take two years, *period!* Okay, it won't, really, but it's better to underpromise and overdeliver, right? Get a few months into it and it will be as much fun as making your teeth a brighter shade of white: that comes from repeated use of a battery-operated toothbrush and the right "performance enhancers," doesn't it?

Sure, okay, you say. This is all true; it's hardly rocket science. I know all of this anyway. It's just that I don't know if any of it will work for *me*. After all, I might have bad genes. With all of the recent hype over biogenetics and how that makes a difference, for either good or bad, people do or don't do all sorts of things. Maybe this is where you are. All I ask is this: "Who will you put your money on? The you with great genes on a daily diet of dollar burgers, never again making it to the gym, or the you, with not-so-great genes, who refuses to miss a workout and continues to eat and supplement like a champion? Are you still skeptical? I bet you're not. Anyway, now you know what this book is all about!

Continuing on into the book, you will meet a few characters. One is my five-hundred-and-then-some-year-old Ponce DeLeon, who got the idea of getting out of Leon before it got to him. He took with him his bride, Ms. D (never to be confused with MD) and made a pact with her never to age right on schedule, as all of their friends, relatives, and neighbors were doing back in the old country. The only good thing about that "growing old gracefully" hokum was that it was simple to promise the king fifty barrels of Fountain of Youth water to cure the problem. That got them the funding for the voyage. Need I say that they never returned?

You will meet other characters too. If you like Rocky (Sly Stallone) and *his* Ms. D, Adrian (Talia Shire), think Jack LaLanne is the tenth of the wonder of the world, still get a smile over aerobic mistress Jane Fonda going after poverty or something similar, and think the whole world ought to be looking seriously at middle-aged Olympic wonder woman Dara Torres, you just might enjoy yourself. These people all help make the major points about what you need to take much more seriously than the media. But be careful: by the time you get to the epilogue, you just might see your lifelong friends from the Normal Majority in a very different light. And that, my friends, just may be scary. But it is exactly what's *has* to happen if you're going to make a permanent change.

Conclusion

Do start thinking of yourself as a health-conscious person instead of a Health Nut.
Don't take the Normal Majority seriously.

2

We Know More Than the Doctors Do

If the assertion in this chapter title hasn't made you want to see all of the copies of this book burned and Ms. D and me turned over to the House Un-American Activities (a modern day Spanish Inquisition), there's hope. To put your mind at rest, we do know that when it comes to procedures such as performing surgery and setting bones, the doctors do know more. But when it comes to remaining a virtual (biological) pre-thirty-something for a very, very long time, we think that you should hear us out. You *are* interested in that, aren't you?

Ms.D and I expect you are, but we also know that some folks will be unable or unwilling to listen. If that's you, you may be saying that it's because neither of us has a PhD, or even an MD. As if having neither of these isn't enough, we haven't even been Oprah's personal trainers! So, then, what right could we possibly have to tell you anything?

We know how you feel. There is someone trying to convince someone of something every minute on the Internet. We expect your Inbox is as crowded with junk mail as ours. But we do hope you'll hear us out anyway. After all, we're both five hundred years old and still looking great in our Speedo swimming suits every summer on the beach. That should count for something, don't you think?

First consider the possibility, though, that your initial resistance to us has a lot, and I mean a whole lot, to do with the sensible conviction that none of us is getting any younger, and that is just the way it is. Therefore, whether Ms. D and I are high-degreed, world renowned authorities on health or the great Jack LaLanne himself, we are not to be taken seriously. Rather, we should be relegated to the "lucky" category, having been blessed with good genes. Besides, believing that diet, exercise, and supplementation will actually work makes you nothing more than a Health Nut.

This brings us to the second big objection. You may believe that, when it comes to matters of health, a good American should say: "That is what we have doctors for, not self-proclaimed authorities. Mds are the ones who know how we all should live. That's what they've been trained for, and that's why we all should listen to them, including you and your Ms. D. And, as living proof that they're right, they drive two Mercedes, which is a lot better than your crummy little Audi."

To put it simply, anyone who even jokingly says that he or she knows more than doctors do is believed to be arrogant. Okay. We think you might be right. MDs truly do have some good things to say, which, if followed, will keep you alive longer than if you never consulted with them. But I'll bet we're in better shape than they are; and I'll bet that we're more interested in getting you to 140—yes 140—years old than all of them are. After all, the Normal Majority whom they so fastidiously serve would have a real problem with the American Medical Association if anyone in it started coming up with those kinds of professional aspirations.

With that, you may strongly agree and think that maybe, just maybe, there might be something of value in what we're up to. If so, it may make you say, "Wow, you really do look great. If I hadn't seen your driver's license, I never would have believed your age. How did you do it?" Then you will take out your notepad and ask where we will be lecturing. The idea is that we must have something important to say—something that could transform your life.

That's what you *could* do. But chances are that you won't, largely because you *can't*. If you actually did show up at the club every day, you might think you are a closeted Health Nut. So instead, you will start wondering about our genes. That's the politically correct thing to do in situations like this. Without a very extraordinary set of genes, not even five hundred years of diet, supplementation, and daily workouts would have paid off, or so you are expected to believe. In other words, we wouldn't look the way we do primarily because of anything we did. Rather, it would be because of how we were born. Before even hearing us out, you will then conclude that we have nothing very important to say.

Believe as you will, but Ms. D and I, a grad-school faculty of two, think you ought to reconsider for the following reasons:

- ❖ First, we know what we've done for the last five hundred years, and we've been successful at it.
- ❖ Second, we did start up the first health club and have seen results in those who listened to us.
- ❖ Third, we've seen myriads of folks who didn't stick with their diet, exercise, and supplementation for more than the standard ninety-day period, claiming afterward that our program didn't work.
- ❖ Fourth, neither you nor we have graduate degrees in genetics, and none of us regularly has lunch with those who do.

These four things are far more real to us than the standard gene explanation when it comes to superlative healthiness. We hope they will be to you as well. But maybe you're still skeptical. But perhaps our basic humanity will make that go away.

We only advise people to do what we ourselves do. That makes us able to predict how long it will take to see results if a person keeps at it. Therefore, we have very little need for a questionable gene theory. We just think it's little more than justification for still being pear-shaped after six months of "consistent" working out—a la cell phone conversations between sets, and days off for muscle recovery, and missed sessions because of "pressing family or business matters." Gene theory says, "It's not me that keeps me looking dumpy, it's my body chemistry." Friends, in all of our centuries as health club owners, we have never (except once or twice, maybe) seen anyone stay love-handled after six months of truly consistent workouts, dieting, and supplementing.

That's why we think that if you aren't benefiting from what we're recommending, you aren't investing enough of yourself every day. In fact, you're probably only going through the motions when you feel like it—possibly twice a week, assuming you're not too sore or too busy. True or false? *You* be the judge. I know there are very few folks who really can't benefit from diet, supplementation, and exercise. But is this really you?

If going up twenty pounds in a week doesn't sound like you, you may be admitting to being a secret "on again, off again" type. At the very least, you may know that this is the reason none of your New Years' resolutions have worked out. You've made them numerous times, and by March 15 you've found yourself almost completely back to the same old habits. That's how the Adkins diet went by the wayside ... *after* the Mayo diet, *after* the Beverly Hills protein plan, *after* the biweekly visits to the trainer, and finally *after* the daily ride on the exercycle, which now gathers dust in the garage.

So when it comes to you, you will say to yourself, "I should have stuck with it," or "If only I had done it more." We agree, of course, but stop with the remorse. It's a sad waste of time and energy. Just remember that you are not gaining any time since your last birthday and that guilt saps your muscle power. Thus, you need to drop the dreary attitudes *immediately.* In other words, skip the guilt and fear that one more time won't be any different. Friends, it might. *Doubt your doubts and get over to the health club!*

What you should do is simply start again today with resolve to be as regular at it as you are about brushing your teeth. (You never thought of it that way before, did you?) Sign up at the club and then actually do your first workout, and block off a set time every day for the same thing. After that, you can go shopping to get your mega-multivitamins, your low-fat, low-carb foods, and a book on healthy cooking. You might even want to check out Jane Fonda's website. If that sounds too simple to be effective, or if it makes you want to check with your MD to see if sitting with a bag of potato chips in front of your laptop might not be better, act your age! (No one like us ever told you to do that, did they?) In other words, just stop the excuse-making and doctor worship, and get on with the *right* things.

Friends, training as if you were going out for the swimming team in high school (which is what this is like) won't kill you, wear you out, or turn you into a fanatic. It doesn't do any of those things. We don't even think your real MD will tell you that it does, though the one in your head might. If you had been doing it regularly every day for twelve months (to say nothing of five hundred years) you would know what we mean. It's the same with brushing your teeth more than once per day: it won't take off tooth enamel! That was another lunacy held by many not too long ago.

Living athletically has a regenerative effect. It produces energy and creates a spirit of calm optimism, hardly the frenzy associated with bodybuilders back in the fifties, who were all supposed to be compulsive and subject to becoming muscle-bound. Very, very seldom does this happen, but it can; we have seen one athlete who fit this mold. So our critics are not entirely wrong. It's just that their fears cause phobias that keep most people from doing the things that are really best for them.

Exercises like swimming, running, cycling, and higher-repetition weightlifting (twelve reps and up), pumps blood through the tissues, which:

- ❖ Eliminates toxins
- ❖ Keeps the veins from clogging up
- ❖ Keeps the muscles toned
- ❖ Oxygenates the whole body
- ❖ Creates an endorphin-like effect
- ❖ Elevates your mood
- ❖ Puts a lift in your step

If fueled by low-fat, low-carb eating and adequate supplementation, it causes tissue growth, replenishing whatever has been lost due to exertion or stress. In other words, it *really is good for you* and really does have invigoratingly pleasant effects.

The fact that people do not let this influence their actions is somewhat baffling to Ms. D and me. For literally decades (and figurative centuries), we have derived daily benefit from daily exercise, supplementation, and low-fat, low-carb eating. Yet most people, the Normal Majority, deeply believe that living in this way will most certainly drain all of the energy out of you, causing irreversible tissue loss, decreased longevity, and exhaustion. We have referred to this elsewhere as "wearout," an imaginary physical phenomenon that has nothing to do with the disappointment and despair (psychological trouble) associated with corporate America's burnout.

Wearout, the feared result of really working out in a GOFHW manner, has to do with exhausting energy reserves and tissues. This is nothing but an old wives' tale. Sadly, nothing could be further from the truth. All you need to do is to see a picture of Jack LaLanne after seventy years of it. He was born in 1914! Google him if you don't believe me.

Being fortunate enough to have been born into the great United States, we think you owe it to yourself to start thinking and start living athletically. That is far different than living the "take it easy," or "have a great day" American good life with timeouts for McDonald's, "Miller Heavy" (not Lite), and an every other Saturday afternoon softball game, (maybe). You should start today.

You ought to hang in there with all of the other "Health Nuts" like us. That will make a noticeable difference in you in six months, which will be followed by a transformational one in twenty-four months. After thirty-six months, your doctor will be envious. This *will* (not may) happen even if everyone you know says you're too old to start, or that they've "been there, done that." Just remember, these folks never did anything beyond the first ninety days, and maybe never even after the first fifteen.

If you're not laughing, this book may not be for you. Or you may still be taking the Normal Majority too seriously. That is understandable. After all you're still a newbie! And they really do think they know everything—especially the young ones—even a whole lot more than the doctors. What's more is that they're you're good buds, so they must be right, right?

Okay, now you're cracking up. If you know they aren't always right, then you're really taking the first step to experiencing a whole new world. Are you still with us? Hope so!

Conclusion

Do take Modern Medicine advances seriously.
Don't let it keep you from being all that you can be.

3

Is Turning Back the Clock Politically Incorrect?

Most adults really don't want to get older. Some may, if they think that clout comes with years, but most dream of being younger or staying at the age they are at forever. Thanks to all of the wonders of modern science, that just might really be possible. Of course, the younger we are, the more desirable this is.

Stopping the clock nowadays seems to be doable. Turning it back? Well … maybe by next year, who knows? It is best to work with what seems real. So stop the clock, and do it now—the earlier the better. This is where most of us are, largely because of what's been done to arrest cancer, to slow down its progression.

Slowing down a dread disease like cancer is supposed to give you a few more good years. Of course, they may not be as good as they were before, but they will be better than the regression Mom and Dad may have experienced. Yet that is what is supposed to happen when (not *if*) you get to the nursing home. This is where you go to die, which means losing all of your faculties one by one, including your mind. Putting that whole sad inevitability off for ten years or so is what makes the nausea of chemo worth it.

Today, most people believe that you can slow down degeneration. In other words, you can get cancer with its death sentence but know that with enough radiation and therapy, you can pretty much stop the whole deterioration process and resume a normal life—for a while longer at least. Sometimes you even get cured! Therefore, the same should probably go for remaining forty-five a whole lot longer, if only one did the right things before the cancer. That's generally how the hopeful thinking goes.

But to have this occur, how does one stop the clock during middle age? Clearly, it's not with drugs, as might be the case for a cancer diagnosis in your later sixties. Instead, it's with lifestyle changes. Then you get on a low-fat, low-carb diet, along with a mandatory daily exercise routine fortified with some mega-multivitamins and herbs. Everybody knows that will work, don't they?

"Well ... maybe everyone does, but it's pretty risky actually pulling this off." Thus saith the Normal Majority. But maybe not everyone is even a little bit sure. We know that there are an awful lot of folks who still say, "I don't know that diet, exercise, and supplements really do their thing." So quite a bit of skepticism is always to be expected when it comes to working out, dieting, and taking supplements. The same goes for a skepticism about being in touch with yourself, which makes you rely heavily on your doctor.

Before listening to anything we have to say, it's only natural to first see if you're healthy enough to live healthily. So it's only prudent to make that doctor appointment. That's the prevalent thinking, at least. Thus, you will go to him or her, and there's no two ways about it. We know. So hurry up and get it over with. Nothing good will happen until you start doing something consistently with the same regularity as you brush your teeth; and you won't do anything until you get your good-to-go stamp. So do what you must and have your doctor's receptionist put you on the calendar.

All we ask is that you think about how to ask the right questions before you get there. Here are a couple of suggestions:

- ❖ Doctor (who presumably doesn't have a first name), is it okay if I do some preventative healthy living so I don't look the way my parents did when they got close to the end of their days?
- ❖ I was thinking about outdoing Jack LaLanne by the time I get to be ninety-five, and I was wondering if there was anything you knew about me that might make this too dangerous.

Either of these may raise an eyebrow, but they most likely will get a suggestion more helpful than "You'd better be careful at your age." They will also get you a permission slip to start acting in a health-conscious manner, which is what you really wanted, isn't it?

How do we know about your MD? Because an increasing number of doctors are starting to care about preventative health, knowing that this goes hand in hand with diet, supplementation, and working out. That's common knowledge. They also know that their drug-based cures work better on those who are biologically younger (or not as worn out yet), meaning healthier. So if you do catch or get something, your doctor has a far better chance of curing you. Besides, most every major illness nowadays is somehow linked to too much weight, and this is most easily corrected by a regular training program.

In short, the MDs are to some degree on our side, and they ultimately care about you. That means, in spite of what the cynics think, they really do want more than to perform needless operations to pay for their summer house, or to get perky kickbacks from the drug companies. In other words, they are MDs in the end: doctors who are truly doctors.

When we started the first health club back in the sixteenth century, things were not much different than they are today. Everybody back then wanted to live forever too. Everybody also knew that just couldn't happen. They were all as smart as you are in that regard. Just like your grade school teacher said, "People start to die the moment after they're born." They all believed the same: that progressing deterioration further translated into getting hopelessly worse-looking year by year, starting with your thirtieth birthday. That was believed to be no more or less than realistic. Only a child or Health Nut would expect otherwise. Accepting this without complaining was, as it still is, the essence of adulthood. It gets you a card-carrying membership in the Normal Majority association.

We, of course, have trouble with this dignified compliance (gracefully aging) and have been complaining about it for five hundred years. And there are now others who are studying arduously to find ways to turn back the clock. We are all about keeping the dream of a fit-forever USA alive. Hopefully, you'll become part of our quest, using your head about health matters instead of investing any more of your life in always agreeing with the Normal Majority.

Conclusion

Do refuse to deteriorate.
Don't think acting your age is cool.

4

What Is Going On in the US, Really?

How is it that the healthiest country in the world can have billboards encouraging us to do things such as walk up the stairs instead of using the elevator? Doesn't this suggest that we need inspiration for making it up a flight or two from the ground floor? The same goes for pulling weeds. Is this too hard as well? If we aren't pulling our own weeds or raking the leaves right now, who is? Is it the hired help or the homeowners' association? In some instances, maybe, but not that many of us are so lucky. In a healthy nation, how can it be that we are being coaxed into taking the stairs or doing the gardening?

It must be that fewer and fewer of us are doing anything active anymore. Why else? Granted, there are more health club members now than there were ten years ago, but it's questionable whether any of those people have the courage to break a sweat when working out. It's also unclear how many even actually stay with it after the first ninety days. The number of those who sign up is drastically different from the number still with it after a year. In fact, this number decreases in fewer than three months, which is the reason for keeping a sales staff on board.

Yet there are those who last beyond the critical fallout dates. They are generally taken less seriously at the office than their more laid-back counterparts, maybe because being dedicated sounds too gung ho (another variation of Health Nut.) It suggests a set routine, probably on the machines occasionally interspersed with cycling. If there is a pool, the lifting may be augmented with swimming. But seldom are any of the routines weights only. There is still too much fear of becoming a muscle-bound dumb jock. That really would be too high school for the with-it American.

Nowadays, a few folks routinely go about their daily workouts to stay fat free. If they keep their mouths shut about it, they can pursue these indoors without being labeled as Health Nuts. The neighbors can't nail them like they could for jogging ten years ago. So there is some headway. There are more people doing the right things this year in comparison to last. And that is a plus—but it's not good enough.

People have to be incognito when working out. If we're talking about you, you know exactly what we mean. You are probably living next door to the chairperson of the House Committee on Anti-Athleticism, a subcommittee of the Normal Majority, so you "don't run around the block in your underwear," as they call it. That would be the same as hanging your dirty laundry in public.

It would be great to make a statement by running past these friends and neighbors of yours every day at the same time (how Ms. D and I would love it), but you will have enough to do keeping up your workouts without lobbying for a healthier America. So don't you be the one. Rather, stay inside the club or in the pool, on the track or exercycle. That's the only way to avoid criticism for doing the right things. If you don't, opting for being open and honest about it with the wrong folks, you will find that it makes for some unpleasant conversation.

It's a sad commentary on our country, especially considering our astronomical health costs, that the only way to stay at a training routine is to be secretive—secretive about something that would be good for everyone. But that's the way it is, so that's what you should do, unless you have an overabundance of crusader zeal about you.

We, of course, wish things were different. Having a few folks wish you well as you stride past them is somewhat the same as getting cheered like Rocky (assuming you've seen the movie *Rocky I*) running through the streets of New York in preparation for his first big fight. That's what should be happening, along with an ever increasing number of couch potatoes getting off their couches each week. This is exactly what we'd like to see all of the time; that might actually be enough to make everybody stay at it seven days a week. This means doing some GOFHW in spite of rain, snow, "not enough time," and the like.

If it happened that Ms. D's and my efforts got a few folks started on the right track, even just at the club, it would be good. But, good is not awesome, we're sure you would agree. We should all want to see a large percentage of runners in work out shorts and tank tops building up their stamina and bodies, while a smaller percentage of couch potato neighbors applaud in genuinely envious respect. Right now, it's the other way around. The aspiring marathoners get laughed at not only by arrogant couch potato strangers, but also their pear-shaped friends, relatives, and neighbors (their personal Normal Majority!)

We want to see an end to this Health Nut label. It's what makes it possible for the aging normal folks of the Normal Majority to ridicule the Health Nuts as perpetual adolescents. The ones who get the brunt of these put-downs are the very people who not only take care of their own bodies for themselves but very positively affect the health of the people around them. They even cost the insurance companies far less! So it really makes no sense that they get called Health Nut. You would agree with that, wouldn't you?

In-shape people are better to be around; they're more reliable, optimistic, and just plain fun. We aren't even prejudiced in favor of them; they just are. You can see this for yourself, and if you are still a couch potato, we really hope you take notes. You will see that the Health Nuts don't spend as much time in the hospital, if they even ever get there at all. Further, they lack a basic cynicism, with its witch-cackle laughter ("Been puttin' on a little, haven'tcha?" or "Not getting any younger, are ya?", always accompanied by that chilling *heh heh heh*). If you don't know this, you don't know any dedicated healthy people and you probably can't hear your own just-jokings when you are simply being nice, warmly and with kudos, of course, calling your children "Health Nuts," quite often to their face!

This is where things are today. For a healthier country, this must stop before the start of "sometime soon." Every day a health-conscious person has to call himself a Health Nut, or hear that from someone with a forty-two-inch middle, we should all realize that our country is not as good as it should be. The sad result is not only one person's diminished happiness but also the existence of more diabetes, more heart trouble, and more unsightly fat.

No one serious about his or her health can really tolerate these disgusting put-downs from people who ought to know better. That's why there are broken commitments over daily workouts and more friendships that finally get in the way of daily workouts. The former happens when you start acting your age by spending more time with your friends, thereby keeping your critics happy, the latter when you rightly say, "No friend would make me feel bad for doing what is good for me and everyone else, so bon voyage." None of us wants either of these. Yet they happen all of the time.

Why should anyone in this great land object if his best friend or spouse starts working out? After all, weren't we always all about beating everyone else in the Olympics, being the most fit country in the whole world and all that?

MsD and I think that it's at least partly because of misinformed concern. The Normal Majority believes that the Health Nut exerts himself far too much for his own good. That's something that is supposedly sure to lead to a bad end (wearout).

Whether the Normal Majority is really sincere about this or not, it allows them to put on a parent-like concern. They think that by discouraging others from sweating and escalating their heart and respiratory rates, they are helping them prolong their lives. Maybe that's because R & R is what the American good life is all about; and if it's American, it must be as good as it gets. What can explain this absurdity better? Anyway, it exists in the here and now in our country.

Ms. D and I strongly disagree with all of this, of course. We don't think that hard work makes you wear out, but we do believe that a life of ease makes you *rust* out. That's why we love working out. Doing so leads to a good night's rest and more energy the next day (to say nothing of an enviable body). Sadly, those sentiments are not shared by most people, the card-carrying members of the Normal Majority. If they were, they'd be vigorously doing their workouts. Instead, "havin' a great day" and "takin' it easy" are what they're telling themselves and everyone else to be doing. Consequently, the life of R&R is almost universally where things are today.

Without asking everyone we meet (or doing an extensive study), we have to assume that the Normal Majority doesn't know any different. That is, they don't know any better. Rather, they all think that they're either doing the right things or preaching the right things when they're in sync with what the doctor said or with what all of the ads on TV imply—in other words, living pretty much as they were taught to. After all, their parents advocated much the same, and they didn't die early. They both made it to at least seventy-five. So there you have it! How much more justification does a person need?

Clearly 99.999 percent of these folks have become pear-shaped and worn out since their forty-fifth birthday, but presumably there's nothing wrong with that. There's nothing wrong with that because they said so, that is. They all aged right on schedule, so they look pretty much like what you'd expect. Besides, they're okay by medical standards—"doctor said so." So where's the problem, they ask? How common is this nowadays?

The Normal Majority forces you to take it easy on a daily basis. That may not sound reasonable, but that is the way it is. Say "I refuse" when told to "take it easy" and you will see what we mean. Step out of line by talking about an improvement in your regular morning run and you will find yourself in trouble. If that doesn't get you amiably but directly called a Health Nut, it will get you warned against overdoing it. You will then be indirectly encouraged to act your age. All of this is done in your best interest, of course.

The problem is that it results in some strange and upsetting realities—ones that Ms. D and I, at least, are aware of all of the time. You probably are as well. They include, but are not limited to, high blood pressure, overweight, diabetes, stroke, and heart problems. And all of these are on the rise in the world's healthiest country!

Because of this need to eradicate exertion from the American good life, the great USA has become predominantly populated by overweight and flabby citizens. Even kids in their early teens are flabby and in need of treatment for cholesterol, heart trouble, and diabetes. Walk on a busy street and you'll see hardly anyone without some excess baggage above their belt line. Granted, in LA and New York, this may not be as much the norm, but it *still* is the norm even in those places. Now it has even spread to the UK! How did this happen? When did it happen and why? Surely there must have been a time when it wasn't as prevalent, wouldn't you think?

Historically, we can't be sure, even if we are five hundred years old. Things like sags and dumpiness creep up over time. All we know is that these conditions have been increasing with each half decade along with a general slowing down of everything as people approach sixty-five—or is it eighty-five nowadays? Maybe that's not the way it always was, but for sure that's the way it is now, and that's what we have all come to expect here in the United States.

Only Health Nuts like Ms. D and I would protest. And how absurd is that? When people do not make it to forty-five in other places around the globe, and when here, more people have fewer life-threatening things wrong with them, there is no right to complain, right? Okay, we agree a little. We're fortunate as a nation. But is that as good as it should be allowed to get? Is it good enough for you?

Granted, very few of us suffer from malnutrition and the devastation of disease. In other words, we are not affected by the ills that plague other parts of the world. For this, we should be grateful. As a result of the AMA and advances in medical science, more people here are able to live longer than ever before. That is good, but you have to decide whether you might want more. If you don't, you'll fit right in. The Normal Majority will accept you wholeheartedly. They'll let you in. Maybe the psychological reassurance itself of being one of *them* will add a decade or so to your golden years. But Ms. D and I wonder how you can look in the mirror and say, "That's good enough for me and for my Ms. D or Ponce."

The crucial thing to keep in mind is that in reality the American good life is not like the really good life we're promoting. Our good life is anything but the life of ease and luxury (R&R without end). Rather, it's a life of supplementation and low-fat, low-carb living with more than a touch of athletic dedication thrown in on the side. That's the set of ingredients needed for making people optimally healthy at any age.

But you may object and say, "Who wants to train like this at *my* age?" The quick answer is, "I'll bet you do, and there are a growing number of those who feel the same." You may still need to ask, "Will I make it?" followed by a cynical witch cackle, something like that bad old *heh heh heh.* My answer to you: "Ditch the Normal Majority while working to get biologically younger."

You do have this option, in case you didn't know. Things are changing. That's part of what is going on here in the great USA, the land of the free and the home of the brave, just like it's always been. It's just that a lot of people here still don't know that they can take charge of their own healthiness and really make their lives better … lives that really can last far longer.

People are working on longevity projects as you read. Things really are evolving, which means that you can do more to determine your own destiny. You have choices, options. That's in the here and now alongside the locked-in program of aging right on schedule—the one that the Normal Majority keeps insisting you be part of. All you have to do is to say no to them, while saying yes to us.

Conclusion

Do work out, diet, and supplement to be healthy.
Don't think this makes you "nuts."

5

Starting Is Less Important Than Continuing

Ms. D and I see new people starting at the club all of the time. Unfortunately, this is starting over again in almost all cases, meaning that the previous starts have all bombed out. Nevertheless, a new beginning is a big deal. It's as if this time, for some reason, everything is going to be different. And maybe it will be. A newly hailed fitness guru (like even us, maybe) in a new book may approach the whole topic in a more poignant fashion, which just may do the trick. If so, the enthusiasm takes hold, making everything seem different. That's good. But what's troubling is that even this new optimism seldom lasts for six months, and it is generally completely gone after only three.

We see these mature newbies starting out again, generally this time with a trainer. Maybe they figure that trying it on their own before was what caused their failure. Perhaps that was true. But actually, a $20-per-hour trainer shouldn't be necessary, and they should know this. All a newbie has to do is carry a $19.95 book (like this one) and refer to it whenever he or she gets stuck. Unfortunately, that almost never happens. This suggests that being told what to do is apparently more essential than merely reading paragraphs on the page.

The supposedly essential prod typically comes from someone who is in pretty good athletic shape. This means a *relatively* fat-free person who is certainly less dumpy than the one asking for help. And he or she is well equipped with a clip board to keep track of what's being done. This is nothing very monumental, but it's presumably better than working all by yourself. Granted, you could keep track of how many reps you did on each machine yourself, but the question is, "Would you?" Apparently the answer often is, "I don't trust myself with something like that. That's how I failed the last time."

Therefore, you conclude that a trainer is what you need if you really want to see changes. And there may be some truth to this. After all, Oprah has a trainer, and that presumably helps. Besides, there are signs at the health club saying "What you may just need is a push (from one of our trainers)," and the like. So getting help may make some sense.

Personally, Ms. D and I think that trainers ultimately do neither harm nor good. But we're big believers in self-determination. We think you should tough it out on your own, simply remembering that you owe eight reps on the press machine, ten on leg press, twelve on the triceps push-down, and a half hour of cycling today, just like you did yesterday. Thinking of it that way, as a standard payment, takes away the need for any great push. You just have to make good on your obligation, kind of like paying the checkout person at the grocery store.

Whether they are worth their salt or not, most trainers run their course after a month or so. That's mostly because they cost a lot, even with the thirty-session package deal, and are seldom available when you need to do your workout. Thus you not only have to pay more than you can afford, but must also adapt to *their* schedule. Neither of these is good for you. Oprah may have money to burn and a relatively flexible schedule, but the average person does not.

By in large, health club trainers aren't very inspiring. That's unfortunate, though not entirely their fault because they wear two hats. They also do the marketing for the club, which they may feel is more important (commissions, pressure from the club owner, etc). Most likely, they aren't one tenth as good as the self-proclaimed guru who wrote your book (not us … someone else with bigger biceps or whatever), though there are exceptions.

What seems most true is that reading this book over and over (as you should) is not a very popular way to go when it comes to working out. It's as if reading is a "been there, done that" type of thing once you get to the last page. In other words, people would rather have personal support when it comes to this type of thing. Unfortunately, your author can't be right there with you.

Trainers are right there, however, and they can say things that you might not be inclined to say to yourself or hear from the author, who should be, but probably is not, inside your head. Thus, giving you an appropriate, very real "guts it out" or "press harder" could be what a trainer's good for beyond the first week of tutorials on the machines. The same goes for pep talks about how to make it through the tough times, what to eat and when, and how to supplement intelligently. But this almost never happens, even if the trainers themselves would like it to. If it did, they know they might get into trouble with their bosses, the club owners, at the very least.

Remember that personal trainers are accountable to the club owners, who think that everyone should be going through the motions to make the gym floor look safe for new prospects coming through on tour. (Have to make things look hospitable to the newbies, right?) Besides, they all remember those "take it easy" signs that used to be all over: "don't breathe hard; don't perspire." You know which ones we mean. Granted, they may no longer be as prevalent, but the Normal Majority will never forget them and expects that club owners are mature, normal folks who keep things safe for everyone—thereby earning them the right to stay in business. Anyway, the club has got to stay safely attractive if it's going to stay profitable and avoid getting a bad name from the Normal Majority, something that will get it shut down.

That's the biggest reason trainers don't say anything dynamic to anyone, which sadly includes all those who may be in need of just that. Nevertheless, they provide positive reinforcement for whatever got you started in the first place— namely the guru who wrote your book. They do this without even knowing that you bought a book in the first place; after all, you never told him or her, did you? Nevertheless, the trainer is right there as a kind of extension of the author.

Keeping you showing up is what trainers have to do as a function of customer retention, converting your month-to-month agreement into a year-long contract. That's actually not all that bad, though, really, because sticking with it is nine-tenths of the fitness battle. You'll just have to hope that nature spurs you on when needed and hangs in there with you when the trainer's no longer there.

Teaching you all about the machines is pretty much what trainers do almost universally and exclusively. They can be counted on for that. All of them have professional certificates which says they know *quite a bit about this stuff.* Unfortunately, that's where their expertise stops. And that, by the way, is probably the best reason for you to stop working with them as soon as you have learned what you need to for your fitness objectives. You need the money that they cost to get through the transition from grocery store food to organic food and to cover supplement expenses, which you are not yet accustomed to. Exceptional trainers like Burgess Meredith's character in *Rocky I* are a whole different animal, as we'll discuss later. If yours is like this, you should hang onto him or her.

One thing most trainers almost never do is get into diet and supplementation. They may suggest a well-balanced diet, as they can't really get into trouble for this. After all, the three balanced meals from the four food groups without all of the goodies plan has been around forever. The Normal Majority believes in this as well, even if they can't stay away from cheeseburgers, Miller (Heavy), and everything else that screws up a training routine.

You will have these inclinations as well as you turn from a Normal Majority member into a health-conscious human being. You could avoid them by using green tea pills, for example, making your training easier and far more consistent. In other words green tea pills are good, and should be promoted; and they are 100 percent different from severely cutting back Monday through Friday, only to be encouraged to reward yourself for all your hard work with a couple of Arby's now and then—or whatever the Normal Majority thinks you can't live without.

But trainers will never come out and say something like "Have you ever tried a green tea cap right before your workout and then a couple of times throughout the day? Those will escalate your whole system, cause the blahs to vanish, curb your appetite, and make you feel great." Trainers will never say anything like this, even if they wouldn't dream of making it through the day without *their* green tea caps. The presumed fear is that they will indirectly encourage an overdose, and that could result in your complaining to the owner. They might lose their jobs, or in absurdly extreme circumstances, you might sue them. Besides, pill recommendations—better known as prescriptions—are only for doctors to do, right? Yup, that's true.

Of course, we don't think an MD will recommend or prescribe green tea caps either. That suggests we shouldn't even bring this up (as we're doing) in black and white. But Ms. D and I think you'll probably make out just fine if you buy an over-the-counter supply of these and then just use your head. (Don't ask the MD if it's okay to think, okay?) They must be pretty safe, right? After all, they are right there in front of you at Walgreens, and there are directions on the bottle. Our favorites are the green tea caps, but maybe there's something else that you will find more enticing—for example, guarana or willow bark.

The blahs, of course, are prevalent when you're starting out. It takes quite a while (figure six months) to get good and to have a workout that's something you look forward to. Green tea caps help you get through this initial period and maintain your daily pace. That's a *must*.

Friends, you absolutely have to stay regular at this workout pace, or you will never make it beyond the fourth week. Getting a little help from your friends, the caplets, is far superior to getting anything from your overstuffed friends, relatives, and family members—believe me! Stay away from them along with their goodies, and keep a bottle of these pills with you at all times.

Of course, green tea caps are pills, and as such, the Normal Majority has a real issue with them. The latest is that they're bad for your liver, as if all of the stuff they push on you is not. The Normal Majority is fond of the absurdity of always eating only "real food," as they call it, drinking all the coffee they need (psychologically, that is), and doing what their bodies tell them to do.

Friends, if you keep this up, your body will scream at you to take a break—a huge break, like for a couple of months or so. Doing all of that is just too hard on it. The erroneous belief is that a couple of cheeseburgers and a steak are safer than morning, afternoon, and evening doses of green tea pills. Same goes for that sixteen-ounce cup of coffee, despite the caffeine, the cost, and perhaps some added syrup with all of its preservatives and white sugar. They're supposedly better than a nice little ten-cent, zero-calorie pill that breaks down almost instantaneously, doing the things you need to push through your routine more efficiently.

Green tea caps really will help you to stay at your routine, which is of primary importance. But you are still going to get raised eyebrows if you confess to taking them. And we're probably going to get on the FBI watch list for recommending them. So let's just keep this all under wraps, okay? They all have their reasons. Some are better than others, though most have never tried what we're talking about.

Your critics' thinking goes like this: coffee is better because it's been around for a long time, not like the risky new little pill. Besides, real people (card-carrying members of the Normal Majority) don't have any trouble ingesting it, so where's the problem? Besides, again, the FDA thinks it's A-OK, just like cheeseburgers and all of the other real food you can buy at the grocery store (which is different from the marginal, to say nothing of overpriced, whole foods you can buy at the co-op). So maybe the coffee and the real snack will slosh around in your stomach while you're exercising, but what else is new? That's life! You experience the same thing getting off the ground in the morning with hash browns, eggs, and bacon, and you're still alive, right? Everybody should accept all of that type of thing as part of what it means to be human, which is not at all the same as being a Health Nut. Oh, brother, (or sister)!

Our problem with all of this goes straight to the core of the issue. That type of "normality" is too hard on you and everyone else. In other words, it's bad, beyond not okay. You belch it; it weights you down; it results in your getting fat. It basically makes you a miserable person to be around. It causes you to spend all of your energy processing it. You need that energy for your workout, pure and simple.

Attempting to digest some heavy grocery store food and a sixteen-ounce coffee while trying to do the machines, followed by cycling, is so difficult that it becomes virtually impossible. It's enough to make you give up long before there's any real benefit from the workouts. That's something we don't want to see happen. You're with us on that, right?

What you should do when you start a new routine is simply tough it out without all of the food in the Normal Majority's dietary prescriptions, staying instead with a low-fat, low-carb diet. This isn't all that easy, because exercise—which you aren't used to as yet—escalates your appetite. But that's what you have to do. If it's any help, you won't have this problem two years down the road.

The caplets make it infinitely easier to say no to those inevitable hunger pangs, and believe me, they're coming. Hoodia is a new helper that you might want to consider; it makes it far easier to stay on course, trusting that things will eventually work out. This means being able to ignore your own inner timeline, otherwise known as being long-suffering, a sorely nonexistent virtue in fast-everything America. In other words, it allows you to hang in there for far longer than you otherwise would. With the caplets, you can do it without the strain of always being tired and hungry.

Given these little wonders of modern science, it is hard for us to accept that people can start dieting, supplementing and exercising, only to quit everything after fewer than ninety days. We understand why they do, but we don't accept it and we don't dwell much on it. It is not okay, and you should believe that. Period. Zero tolerance. Other folks have stuck with it, so why not you? Period.

Ninety days is close to the point where you ought to just be coming into your own. Saying that it's all too hard and then quitting doesn't cut it. Friends, giving in may seem normal and commonplace, generally with some mature-sounding justification such as not having the time for such frivolity—but it's not something you can allow for yourself.

If you want to look different from all of the other folks on the block, and we assume you do, you must dare to be different. That means hanging in there when it seems only reasonable to quit. Again, the little green pills will help. They will make what I'm saying seem far more do-able.

As an aside, Ms. D and I are admittedly having a great amount of trouble with quick fixes in the form of new wonder-of-modern-science pills that anyone can hear about in the standard TV commercial. Thus, some of the Normal Majority will say that we're no better than them, pushing our little supposedly okay pills. Well, they may have a point.

But if you have a little brown bag (a bag you're supposed to dutifully present to your MD, when she or he is trying to figure what drug to put you on) containing our pills and a little plastic bag filled with standard pharmaceutical, big-drug-company meds, we think you'll fare better with ours (even if the MD doesn't think they're all that necessary). That's because ours don't have high costs or side effects or the potential to cause other unhappy complications. Furthermore, they don't screw up the real medicines (that is, there are almost no drug interaction difficulties). Nevertheless, you're right; we're pushin' just like the MDs, the advertising folks at the drug companies, and the bad guys with the hard stuff on the street.

We live in a fast-everything culture. Fast communication via the Internet has replaced snail mail. Fast food is on nearly every major intersection. Drive into McDonalds, eat, and throw away the containers. Much easier and quicker than washing dishes after cooking, wouldn't you agree? There are quick cures for serious problems that have been a long while in the making. Take the latest pill when diet and exercise don't work because *we* don't work anyway. Just ask your doctor if the new pill is right for you. And if you've just done that, maybe that's because you decided that diet and exercise didn't work.

Wonder why diet and exercise didn't work? We don't. They didn't work *fast* enough for you, which really means you didn't hang in there long enough and put enough of yourself into them. If only you'd had some green tea caps. Trust me; this all gets more fun and effective with time. You just have to hang in there long after the sensible folks have decided to hang it up.

Anyone who's trained for a state meet or a Miss America contest back in high school knows what it took. It took hours and hours of work—hours and hours each day. It took a number of years as well. Some of the really good athletes even trained in grade school, long before they ever got to junior high. Their training was rigorous. But their hours were hard only for the first few months, or maybe not even that long. After that, the routine became part of them; then they were on cruise control, so to speak, always poised for times when they got those special spurts. That's when it all became fun, when it no longer made sense to call it work in the sense of pure drudgery ("Uff da," as they say in Minnesota).

People who know this have no trouble getting back into a healthy routine and staying with it. People who don't know it will have to work extra hard to get that first experience. That's the biggest reason to stay away from the folks who can't help putting you down. They add insult (discouragement) to injury (sore muscles). It's also the best reason for getting some green tea caps.

You know that you need to be doing something on a daily basis that will build your health. It should be a combination of cycling, running, or swimming and lifting weights, in conjunction with proper diet and supplements. The combination will give you muscle tone along with cardiovascular health. Is there anyone who would disagree that two years of never missing a day at this regimen would probably ensure overall healthiness, as well as attractiveness to die for? That it would dramatically enhance the quality of your life? That's all it takes—not stopping any of it once you've started. Does this really not make sense to anyone?

Conclusion

Do start again, this time using something like green tea caps. *Don't* think of healthiness as anything different from brushing your teeth.

6

The Intimate Wet Blanket

You would think that being in super shape or even just megahealthy would be a turn-on in a marriage. We all want to be proud of our spouses. We all want them to be love-handle free. We all want them to feel great. Everyone wants the best for the people they're close to. Surely no one can disagree with this, right?

So why all the fuss when one spouse makes an announcement that he or she is going to be doing a regular diet, exercise, and supplementation routine from now until he or she dies? If you are rolling your eyes right now, you are a wet blanket.

A wet blanket is what you put on a flame the size of a small campfire to kill it. Clearly it's not big enough to quench a blazing forest, but it will work on the standard hand-warmer variety. The campfire is the size of the flame we have when we start thinking that it's time to do something in preparation for the summer. Because we want to look good on the beach (or just want to lose the too-many-Christmas-cookies-excess), we make the breakfast announcement: "I'm going on green tea, skipping lunch, and running five miles before dinner starting today … so … want to join me?" If you are married to a wet blanket, this will not get a good reception.

A wet blanket will say, "No, dear, you go ahead if you like," and nothing more. This may sound polite, but behind this niceness is a spouse who is really saying, "I'm too adult (mature) to care about being the stud or the beach bunny." The implication is that "Dear" should be beyond this by now as well. After all, this type of thing might have been okay in extreme moderation when you were both sixteen, but now with PTA, church council, raising the kids, chairing the homeowners' association, and the like, there just isn't enough time for such a frivolous second childhood.

In theory, if aspiring athletes did a better job of getting their spouses on their side, they would start off differently. What they *should* come up with is something like "Maybe we should both start getting with some New Age healthiness. What do you think? After all, we don't like the way our neighbors look, so we should do something before it's too late, wouldn't you agree?" This approach would have a better chance of working, all other things being equal. It would have an even better one if they had been commenting on how awful the neighbors look or imagining what these folks would look like at the beach.

Spouses who want to do anything arduous know that it is essential to have their Ponce or Ms. D on board. They will (or should) be very interested in forming a pact. That's what Ms. D and I did five hundred years ago so that we would stay nice looking for each other. We didn't want to become like everyone else around us. (By the way, they all looked worse back then, as there was a lot of disease and indigestion, too much bread, tons of red meat, no health clubs, no exercycles, no swimming pools, and for *sure* no supplements. And their teeth were yellow. So forget what you see in the movies.) That made it infinitely easier to stick with everything we've been into ever since.

An approach like this—the opposite of wetblanketness, where only one spouse is gung ho—results in mutual support. In this case, Mr. and Ms. Johnson don't want to look like either of the Joneses and will do anything to keep that from happening. Friends, if you really don't like the way the people next door look, this is the way to go. You and your spouse can start doing laps around the block or cycling every evening after dinner, thereby knowing that you'll never end up like your neighbors, who never do anything. What's even better is that you can have fun lying to them about the real reason for doing it at all. You can do the good old "The MD said we've got to start watching it." It works every time. That will make life easier than telling the truth, which would go something like: "No way are we going to pork out and end up looking like you guys!"

Working out together is far safer for your marriage. If only one of you wants to look really good, the result is the wet blanket syndrome, generally at a very unconscious level. One person makes a decision to radically improve, but the other is either unready to do so or is uneasy with the motivations of the other. Unspoken questions such as "Doesn't she or he love me the way that I am?" create a problem right from the start. These concerns may never be fully articulated, though they will exert a powerful influence.

The naïve assumption is that wifey will be thrilled that hubby is finally on his way to losing the love handles, or vice versa. This is rarely the case. When one starts getting in shape, the other starts feeling guilty or uptight. It's far more realistic to predict that one spouse's couch potato syndrome will prevail and thoroughly discourage the other. Then the workouts stop, causing the Health Nut to say something like, "Been there, done that—now back to acting my age. Sorry for the inconvenience." This is when self-acceptance finally takes over, so both can comfortably grow old together, go back to aging right on schedule and growing old gracefully.

Obviously, no one really wins in this situation. On the surface it appears that the couch potato does, but they both unconsciously agree to settle for less, mellowing out with time. Then their golden years become contented instead of contentious, which makes all of their friends, relatives, and neighbors ecstatic. The Normal Majority thinks that this is the ultimate in adjustment—the reward for years of sticking with the same person for better (love handles included) or for worse, and all that.

The Normal Majority looking in from the outside will respect them for sticking it out. That will be the case even if it's clear that they have endured each other with a stiff upper lip. This is what gets them all of the oooohs, ahhs, and applause at their anniversary celebrations. They have endured it all forever. But we think this is only the sad consolation for what they could have had if they had made the sacrifices necessary to allow for trimmer versions of each other.

None of this is operative in the case of the couple that refuses to ever become like the neighbors. That solidarity (you and me against them) may get them called Health Nut when they're always running around the block, but enduring that from couch potato critics shouldn't be too difficult. All that the Johnsons have to do is to watch the Joneses get dumpier by the month and make their snide comments in private. In other words, this all can be rather fun if you don't mind feeling guilty about being such a one-upper. Ms. D and I, of course, say, "Go for it," as feeling superior is far better than feeling like a Health Nut just because the neighbors think you should feel that way.

Whenever a husband and wife side with each other against couch potatoes like the Joneses, other good things follow. For example, they may develop a yen for together time in the form of a joint trip to the club five out of the seven days of the week. Granted, this is hardly the same as vacationing in Cancun, but it is far superior to watching summer reruns together, or even playing cribbage with a couple of Miller Heavies. In short, where there is no wet blanket there is a good chance of people staying with their training programs and maybe even loving each other all the more. That's far better than what typically goes on.

If people are doing anything at all without this spousal teamwork, it's largely because a doctor has said they should. It may be that more MDs are advocating a diet, supplementation, and exercise regime. But we don't think that what they are now generally doing is very effective. Their advice still sounds too much like something that might appear as a helpful tip on the AARP website: "Do a little walking every day and cut down on the goodies" and all that. At least that's how it registers inside their patients' heads. People don't ever really get turned on by this, regardless of how mature it is supposed to be.

Then too, "You'd better lose fifty pounds by Christmas or you won't live to trim the tree" is not very good either. That's a Doctor Threat. People often won't go for this either, though it is taken more seriously and is thus more effective. It's just that the same old habits come right back as soon as you think you're out of the danger zone. But you can use this as a way to buy off your critics, assuming you can't think of anything else. It will keep you out of the Health Nut category long enough for them to get critical of someone else. Then you're *not* safe unless you keep at it well past the crucial point where you start really looking good.

Assuming you can actually do it in the first place, doing it for Doctor won't transform you forever or, to be more precise, for the rest of your life. The weight either doesn't come off, or if it does for while, it comes right back on. If you want to be forever fit, or beach ready every summer, you must admit that that's what you want and *go* for it.

You need to pursue it for your own reasons, preferably for the way you look in the mirror and to your own Ms. D or Ponce. Those are the best reasons we can think of. Those have worked for us and continue to work. This kind of motivation will help immeasurably because you don't ever want to look like the folks next door.

Once you have a deep desire like this, after having gotten over believing it's too much like getting the date you really wanted for homecoming, you don't need to first ask for a doctor's permission. Of course, you could ask what you should do to get rid of something like your pesky tendinitis in the shortest amount of time. That's actually a good question, if you have pain you don't think should be there.

But that is not the same as asking: "Am I too old or too unhealthy to be starting out on a diet, exercise, and supplementation routine?" That, in our judgment, is *not* a question for your MD. It's like asking: "Am I healthy enough to be acting healthy?" Okay, if you're *really* ill, maybe you should ask. But is that really you? In other words, do you want to be cured, or do you want a permission slip for the equivalent of permanent disability?

Doctors are all for getting you well enough to live your life. They are for putting a cast on your arm, giving you an antibiotic for the bugs you should have been lucky enough to avoid, and for doing the tests that tell you about other things that might be going on beneath your energetic and vibrant surface. They are not Olympic coaches, personal trainers, or even high school coaches. They know how to get you out of the hole but not how to get you winning a marathon on level ground.

So what should you do if you want to stay young forever? You already know, although it can't be said enough. You should:

- ❖ diet,
- ❖ exercise, and
- ❖ supplement wisely.

All you need to remember is that you must do these with the same regularity as brushing your teeth. If you don't, you will find that your only friends will be nice folks who look just as bad as you. That's why you have to start dropping these couch potatoes today (or, in the case of next door neighbors, keep your distance from them). That's just as important as cutting out red meat, morning donuts, and that weekly McDonald's. You have to cut out the friends who call you Health Nut or find it beneath their dignity to joy daily around the block the same as you.

You must stay clear of folks who are afraid of acting like high school kids out for the track team. Not acting their ages puts them on the path to being not okay, which is how the Normal Majority will make them feel. So just drop them like you would the cheeseburgers. Keep them on the Christmas card list if you like, as long as you're too busy to be dropping over for goodies on the holidays.

To really be able to get from your Leon to your Florida fountain in a nice sailboat (with a motor, of course), you will first need your spouse on your side. That means getting him or her out of the wet blanket compulsion. With the right approach, it is possible.

Conclusion

Do get your spouse on board with your health plans.
Don't expect much of yourself until you do.

7

Gee, You're Awesome, Jack LaLanne

There are probably a few other megahealth heroes like Jack LaLanne around today, but we really don't know anything about them. Jack is the number-one marvel, possibly because he has been in the public eye since the late fifties. Every now and then he's back doing an ad for his juicer, or most recently for Target.

Baby boomers can remember him on TV, doing workouts for housewives long before the Jane Fonda videos of the 1970s. But that was nothing compared to what he is today. Granted, his face has an older person's wrinkles and crags, but he is as fit as the athletes on the bodybuilder magazines. Some might even say he's better than them because of his chronological age today, which is ninety-five (born 1914).

The most recent commercial shows footage of him from the 1960s next to today's clip of him holding up a TV on his shoulder. If you think that's nothing, try doing it yourself while still smiling. Until you do, you will not be as impressed by him as you ought to be.

Because his face no longer looks like a young man's, like it did fifty years ago, you may think that megahealth isn't all it's cracked up to be. After all, if it doesn't make you wrinkle free at ninety, what good is it? Sounds rather Normal Majorityish, wouldn't you agree? But you should be aware that there are *no* wrinkles on those abs or pecs.

There are probably some wonder women out there as well. To compare apples to apples, they, too, would have to be ninety (plus a few wrinkles) and in as good or better shape than Dara Torres (the forty-two-year-old swimming wonder woman of the 2008 Olympics). So where are they? Jane Fonda is the one who immediately comes to mind. She still looks great, and she is a spectacular person of the past. However, born in 1937, she is nowhere near Jack's age. So is there anyone else? Maybe you know her. If so, tell her to send us contact information and a photo.

As of right now, we are assuming that life is just unfair. It has somehow inspired only the male sex in the longevity department, and our only example is Jack LaLanne. It has caused him, and him alone, to prove his major point: that the more you keep working at health, the healthier you get. This is a radical assertion even when it comes to more average fitness gurus. Common sense, the collection of the self-evident truths of the Normal Majority, says that keeping up an Olympic workout pace from high school to nursing home (or some much sought-after replacement) just isn't wise. It wears you out—makes you die early. But Jack has shown that his real critics, the better part of the over-forty-five Normal Majority population in this country, are just plain wrong.

When people stand out as peerless, there is always some attempt to whittle them down to size. Hence the fifty-going-on-thirty-five woman is said to have been born with good genes, which is the only reason she still looks good in her jeans. Take these other examples:

- ❖ World class bodybuilder Arnold Schwarzenegger, who "just had a great constitution to start with. If he hadn't, all of that time in the gym never would have paid off" or

- ❖ Dara, "Oh, yeah, she's the lady with the great genes in the Olympics who's breaking swim records like that young guy Michael Phelps, isn't she? She's how old? Boy, she looks great for *that* age" or

- ❖ Jane—"Heck, she still looks pretty good for her age. She must have gotten some good genes from her father, Henry. Of course, there's Peter, too, and movie stars always look great."

That's what the Normal Majority does with exceptional folks. It attributes their success to an exceptional set of genes, as if it's an excuse to explain away a superstar's exceptional nature. Then, and only then, can they feel comfortable with these outstanding individuals.

Your average homme on the plaza (person on the street) has really tried working out and all that, but failed, so the gene theory must surely be right. GOFHW has never worked for him, *only* because of his genetic composition.

It couldn't possibly have been because he never made it past the first ninety days at the club, could it? Oh, no. Surely this must somehow ring true in modern-day America. Don't we always seem to hear "When diet and exercise aren't enough, you should ask your doctor if the new wonder pill is right for you"?

It's as if everybody's really putting out, but none of it is working only because of our constitutions. If nothing seems to be working after a year's worth of effort, there really might be a reason. I have seen an example or two of this, and I suspect that genes caused them. This is profoundly discouraging and may be indicative of either a real problem or one of the side effects of a steroid called prednisone which is severe bloating. But these exceptions aside, our questions remain:

- ❖ How many days do you actually make it to the club?
- ❖ How much effort do you put into each workout?
- ❖ Are your supplements actually enhancing what you do?
- ❖ Is your diet always dollar burgers and French fries?

Maybe the gene theory authorities are right, but it's unlikely, as none of the everyday variety have had any postgrad training in biochemistry. Furthermore, when it comes to looking like an Olympic medal winner, they most likely know nothing of our secret weapon, GOFHW. Or they don't know that this means every day at the same or greater resistances and speeds for at least twenty-four months. For certain, they have never Googled the outstandingly peerless Jack LaLanne.

Schwarzenegger still trains, maybe not as hard anymore, but he still does it. That's why he still looks great. What he did prior to becoming California's governor was grueling, far more so than most ever knew. The people who scoffed at him then apparently knew nothing of his heavy (four hundred-to-five hundred-pound) thirty-hours-per-week weight training or any of the other disciplines that have been part of him since before high school. Or if they knew, it never registered. Thus, he has always been just another superstar with a great set of genes.

The same type of thing goes for attitudes about run-of-the-mill Ms. or Miss Americas on the part of their normal, dumpy counterparts. They think that if she didn't inherit the right chemistry from Mom, the decades of vitamins, exercise, and salads would never have made her so skinny (what some overweight women even dare to call anorexic). She had the advantage over normal people simply by nature. Clearly, if only they had had a few more of these superwoman's genes, they'd look just like her.

C'mon folks, isn't this all rather aggravating? The Normal Majority has such a bad habit of talking down about their betters like this. You don't do this, too, do you?

When it comes to Jack, he would intimidate even the most arrogant average wet blanket. He's in a class all of his own, which no one can come even close to understanding. Sadly, that seems to put him with Martians and other beings from outer space. People who are off the charts like him must have come from the stars (or were possibly hatched). That is really problematic when the country should be studying him and listening to what he has to say instead of relegating him to the freak category.

Our only trouble with Jack is that we really don't know of a time when he wasn't spectacular. In other words, there are no before-and-after photos. According to him, he once was rather average, which is why he just decided to get exceptional and keep at it. But all you see now is what you get, and what you have gotten since the late fifties. It's as if he was born astonishing.

That may be the only drawback to using him as living proof that hard work pays off. Yet he'll tell you that it does; and he'll tell you that it continues to pay off with two hours per day of workouts. (Think about that for every day of the week at your son's or daughter's age, to say nothing of his or your own.)

The saddest part about Jack is that people can't even think about him for more than a few seconds. Their minds shut off right after saying, "Wow, I've never seen anyone actually tear a phone book in half or tow barges while swimming in San Francisco Bay." That's a lot like saying, "Gee, you're amazing, Mr. LaLanne." The bad part about this is that there is nothing that follows, such as, "How does one build up to that point, to say nothing of how can anyone still do that at ninety-five?" Instead, they change the subject, immediately moving on to the weather. It's as if the man doesn't even exist. In that way, Jack LaLanne becomes the out-there, off-the-charts, total freak, someone about whom no one cares in the least.

What does Jack the real man have to say about himself? He thinks that he is as he is because of nothing other than seventy-plus years of keeping at it. What could be more modest? And as he is that modest, he should be even doubly humbling to all of life's spectators. But he isn't. The Normal Majority just doesn't seem to care. Is that because the great Jack LaLanne really isn't important?

Ms. D and I don't think so. We think it's because the Normal Majority is in denial and cannot accept his impressive accomplishments, even going so far as to say they aren't real. According to Jack, you don't start wearing out after high school or college unless you hang it up. You just keep getting better and better. To him, it is simply impossible to wear out by staying active, meaning workouts like his two hours per day. (By the way, we'll settle for one hour, as long you don't miss.) He believes that physical health is like anything else: It gets better with consistent work. This is the opposite of the gut-level conviction of the Normal Majority, who are always telling you, directly or indirectly, to slow down because you're not a teenager anymore.

Take a moment to consider money in place of health. Most people know that if you have money you should take care of it: hold on to it and make it grow. You need it for increasing comfort and retirement in your sunset years. There is never a time when it becomes okay to just let go and let God, unless you are considering joining a monastery or convent. But with health, you are supposed to start cutting back on the effort after your undergrad years. That's how the Normal Majority thinks you conserve yourself, making certain that you make it to seventy-five.

Women have yet to see an age-defying champion like Jack. Perhaps she's about to emerge, having never stopped her preparation for the Olympics or the Ms. America contest after age twenty-one. But as of right now, no one in her nineties holds a candle to LaLanne. Does it follow that none of Jack's secrets work for women? Or does it mean that none of the ladies who watched him on TV back in the late fifties kept at it like he did? Or that all of them tried, but couldn't keep from sliding back after childbearing? Ms. D and I doubt it. She's out there. We just don't know where. We need an octogenarian Dara Torres to remind us that all people are like fine wine, getting better with age. Maybe the real Dara will be just that in another fifty-two years. Who knows? Maybe we just have to wait to find out.

How can you understand Jack's incomprehensible strength and health at ninety-five? If there are no comparables, you can't. You just have to accept it. When you do, you can say, "That's an awesome human being—and if he can do it, so can I." Right now, Jack is still from outer space—far more than just a little different.

Granted, Jack may have had some special breaks in his life, the result of inventing most of the machines you now see at your club or being a TV fitness celebrity (both of which are endorphin boosters, par excellence), but the bulk of his vitality is the result of seventy-plus years of consistent hard work. He simply has hung on when everyone else has hung it up.

As we've said, Jack is more fit than most everyone we know in their thirties! And that's the reason people mimic his every action … Oh: people really do that, don't they? Just like back in the 1960s when the ladies used to watch him as they did their calisthenics, which is what they were called back then? No. No one does! This never happens. Relatively few follow his advice, and almost no one studies him in an attempt to figure out what he did right. How can this be? Are we all brain-dead?

That is the protest of this chapter. As we have said before, no one thinks of LaLanne as a real person. No one says, "He's incredible, and there but for the sad neglect of my own constitution go I." No one hangs his or her head in healthy shame. No one really contemplates him.

We think that should happen. Ms. D even thinks that we could stand a new power figure in Washington. Maybe it should be lieutenant to the surgeon general, or better, just plain personal trainer general. Maybe, too, we could get a right-up-there phenomenon going on including Jane Fonda and Dara Torres as well, making them all joint chiefs of staff. Funny? Maybe it's not. With all of the new concern over preventative health, might this not be just what the doctor (the surgeon general) should be ordering?

While the crowds politely say, "Wow, Jack, you're awesome, but pass me the cheeseburger," the USA gets fatter by the day. It would actually be better if people said, "Jack, we think you're from Neptune, so when is the next ship taking off to get us all back home for a spell?" That's what folks *should* say. Who knows what else they might bring back from Neptune to change everything for the better here on earth?

But unfortunately, they don't and most likely won't. The Normal Majority is all too comfortable being far less than they could be. That's why they don't see this man LaLanne as being as important as MsD and I think he is. Hopefully, you will Google him yourself so you can spend at least ten minutes seeing what we think you should be taking seriously.

Conclusion

Do learn from Jack and his two-hour-per-day workouts.
Don't think that genes alone make the athlete.

8

All About Health Nuts

The N word is a big deal in almost everything. N, of course, means normal, but normal suggests different things to different folks. Normal to a psychologist is one thing; to a climatologist it is something far different. Normal in the case of Normal Majority, the one most relevant to our discussion, means never a weirdo, not a Health Nut.

In our context, if you are normal, you are okay. You pass your annual checkup with no major problems. Your doctor has not gotten uptight about you and is not, therefore, requiring further tests. This suggests no need for medications or involved therapeutic disciplines. Thus, you should be off the hook—okay, or doing well, as they say.

If you have just communicated this passing grade to your Normal Majority friend, relative, or neighbor, you should have been allowed to get on with your day. And that, friends, is precisely what you should have done. But you didn't.

In a fit of boredom (as conversations with the Normal Majority never stray very much beyond the weather) you may have been silly enough to have also confessed to having upped your daily routine at the health club. If only you had quit while you were ahead! But no, you were so happy to have passed the normal tests (blood pressure, pulse rate, maybe even blood work) that you had to blab about your increased reps on the machines at the club or your ability to keep up your morning round-the-block pace for a few more miles; it was a thrill.

We know what you were feeling. It's something that would have been hard to keep inside, and it's only the start of something that will keep getting better and better. But you definitely have kept it under wraps. You didn't. In a spirit of sharing, you had to tell all. Who knows, maybe you could have gotten couch potato Ed out there doing the same things right beside you. He'd be sure to thank you for it tomorrow, right?

No way! All you got was his impression of you as someone who is about to have a problem. You set yourself up as a target for the slow-it-down arrow. Having upped the ante from one to three miles on something as energetic as your morning jog, you should now be put into a marginal category. Just a little cargo shifting the wrong way will capsize your little rowboat. (Normal folks, in comparison, are like massive tankers with adequate compartments for everything they're carrying. Of course, we all know that the *Exxon Valdez* could never tip, right?)

In conversations like the one you may have with this friendly neighbor, you will be told that you have to watch it, especially at your age. Sadly, your Health Nuttiness has already made you look better than your critic does, but that is beside the point. The everyday nature of your exercise routine will supposedly get you in the not too distant future. Only a Health Nut would disagree with an orthodox belief like that. In other words, everyone should know better, but clearly, you do not. You disagree and are told to act you age. Because you need to be told, you get a Health Nut label, kind of like a modern day scarlet letter.

When it comes to the term Health Nut, Ms. D and I get incensed. People doing a daily workout, supplementing, and eating the right foods ought to be respected and encouraged to keep on doing what they're doing, not be told to grow up.

For all practical purposes, in today's bad economy with its astronomical health care costs, it can be said that Health Nuts are even being patriotic. Need we mention that health-conscious people have far fewer reasons to be in the hospital? Therefore, they should not be subjected to debilitating put-downs, even if their running around the block looks clumsy at first.

It isn't easy to begin seriously working out. It's hard, but that doesn't make it absurd or bad, even if we live in an age of comfort and ease. If everyone worked at diet supplementation and working out, the country would be better for it, from greater marital harmony (healthy people relate better than ones who hate what they see in the mirror) to lower overall health care costs. How can what causes those results not be praiseworthy?

I believe that the term Health Nut arises out of the new desire for a surpassingly great quality of life: a desire for more than what the Normal Majority feels should be forthcoming. According to them, we are supposed to be content with increasing fat around the waistline and declining energy with the passing of each birthday. That's what these well-adjusted folks think with their "You can't avoid death and taxes" or "None of us are getting any younger" slogans. Growing old gracefully means welcoming this continual slowdown, which culminates in eternal rest. Staying that way when you're around them allows them to feel comfortable.

Health Nuts, (health-conscious persons, as we would rather they were called) don't see life this way. They think that continuing to work at something will make it better. This includes their health, which they believe can get better the more they work at it. Because they don't share the Normal Majority's aversion to work, they stand out as different—immature and incurably naïve. With trim waistlines and a spring in their step, they stand out as young, which is too much for those who are into growing old gracefully.

The term Health Nut comes from the Normal Majority—the labelers. We even think of some of these authorities on life as being in a class of their own, namely, the Arrogant Anti-Athletic Aristocracy (the AAAA). That may sound a bit harsh until you see them laughing at a newbie trying to get into a running routine. The "What's he trying to prove?" is really unforgivable. If anyone ever did this to a labeler, he or she would call that person rude, which would get you excommunicated, as they said back in the bad old days of sixteenth-century Leon.

The Normal Majority's heroes and heroines are the anchorpeople on the news, who would never be caught dead doing laps around the block. These anchor folks are attractive and in pretty good shape, but not because of what they do. Rather, it's because of what they *don't* do. None of them have any bad habits (that we get to know about). None overeat. None are doctor-bashers, like Ms. D and me once in a while. Nor do they get too upset or too stressed out too often. (Of course, a $250 K-plus salary and notoriety help, but one really shouldn't criticize. That's one of the big causes of major medical problems, so we all believe.)

Yet there isn't anything exceptionally vital about these folks either. For certain, they would not look good modeling for Bowflex equipment or even for their local department store. They just look not bad, and they are very personable, which is supposed to be a touch above good enough. They are living proof that if you don't do anything bad to yourself, the body will take care of itself.

This is really where most of the medical profession and the Normal Majority folks are at. If only they knew how badly some of their supposed minor deviations (the cheeseburgers, the beer, the brats, the weekend pigging out in Vegas, the time in front of the tube, and the like) really are! Surely their heroes and heroines are into these now and then, wouldn't you think? All normal folks are.

Ms. D and I like these CNN-type anchor folks, but think they really aren't doing enough from a health perspective, either for themselves or the Normal Majority who idolize them. That means, we think, they could (and should) have a very positive effect on the whole country. If any of them would confess to a daily mile swim or taking thirty different supplements, the country would be different. Actually, it would be even better if they didn't have to confess at all but instead were open about it, like Oprah. She can get away with dieting, a la acai berries and exercises with her trainer, for … twenty-six months, or was it thirteen? Then everyone, the Normal Majority of admirers that is, would realize that these TV personalities were actually doing something to look the way they do. That would replace the standard view of them as simply lucky enough to have been born the way they are. (Of course, if they 'fessed up, they might be called Health Nuts, and many an eyebrow would rise. So maybe this will never happen. Who can say?)

The people who watch the CNN anchors figure that if they themselves are not seriously ill, they're okay. Granted, these viewers do not look as good as their very personable TV counterparts, but they don't think they are all that far away from it either. Whether they're close or far off the mark, that's how they see themselves, and that's how they demand you think of them. (Try asking them if they haven't been putting on a little lately.) They may have a little extra weight, lack vitality, or be prediabetic, but that's not the same as being seriously badly off, they protest.

Besides, they don't make others uptight by running to the gym or refusing sweets at Christmas. Those are things Health Nuts do. They are normal, they say, which makes them easy to get along with. In their estimation, the world would be better off if the less-together others would simply follow suit.

On the flip page of this category you find our people: the ones called Health Nuts. These are the people who are doing their daily workouts, supplementing intelligently, and closely watching what they eat. Almost always, they are laughed at for acting like this.

What's pathetic is that they sometimes take this to heart. They hear a lot of "You shouldn't be doing that at your age," which may have started as early as when the person just turned thirty-something! That makes them feel endangered even though their standard tests (blood pressure, pulse, heart rate, lung check) come back as exceptional and their bodies are relatively fat free. This ought not to be.

How should they be treated, you ask? With respect, for God's sake! Therefore, we should correct political correctness— and do it now. The current Health Nut label for those who run around the block "in their underwear" should be considered not okay. We've done it before with women's liberation, which made it treason to call women girls. We can do it again with health-conscious people who are now referred to as Health-Nuts.

Friends, we really can get the Normal Majority to drop the attitude. We've done it in the not too distant past, and it wasn't even the first time back then. It's the American thing to do.

The Health Nut underdog should get respect so that she or he can become another Fonda or LaLanne. That's the primary reason to do it, being wholly American in a land of genuinely universal equal opportunity. Everyone should be coolheaded on this issue so that everyone can have the freedom to become as fit as they might like. But that will never happen if people must modify their behavior or keep themselves in secret to avoid the loss of esteem through unkind put-downs. Everyone deserves the freedom to excel at what is good for them. That's what we believe here in our great country.

If the MDs, (never to be confused with Ms. D) were more insistent on diet, exercise, and supplementation, there would also be some significant changes in America. This is another aspect of the problem that needs to be explored. If they did so, they would be influencing from the top down, which would make a world of difference. Living athletically could then be seen as something mature adults can and should be doing, and entirely different view from seeing it as something that only people who don't act their ages can do—a viewpoint MDs are oftentimes guilty of perpetuating in the name of longevity. Telling you to take it easy and slow down is a big part of their way of getting you to seventy, or is it seventy-five nowadays? They will proudly tell you that it used to be sixty-five.

We think things would be way different if the doctors ran during their lunch hours or parked their Mercedes in front of the club every day at the same time and did a respectable workout. But who are we? All we know is that the Normal Majority would never have the courage to call *them* Health Nuts and might even cut their other Health Nut friends some much overdue slack.

If the medical profession were behind daily workouts, there would be respect for the newbie starting out, replacing all the ridicule. If that happened, there would be a dramatic change. More people just might still be at it three months after starting.

But the political side of what we are about should be left to others who are good at just that. So friends, just work at working out, dieting, and supplementing. We know you will have a hard enough time convincing yourself to come to the club every day.

Our suggestion for the politically expert folks is to make Health Nut a politically incorrect term, replacing it with "health-conscious person." That might be a little cumbersome, but it's better than anything else we've got. It's what you should call yourself, catching yourself before you say, "Yup, I'm a Health Nut, I guess" to keep you winning friends and influencing people. Psychologically, refusing to call yourself a Health Nut in private or in public is the absolute first and most important step. The old adage of, "No one will respect you unless you respect yourself," applies here.

The battle starts inside you. It may extend to the people you see every day—your friends, relatives, and neighbors. But it need not, assuming that you keep your mouth shut and do your workouts behind the closed doors of the club. That will spare you all of the arguments and loss of dignity caused by being open, honest, and enlightening with the people you're closest to. That's why we believe in the stiff-upper-lip approach and merely doing your routines in spite of what the Normal Majority has to say.

Of course, we would love to see you relentlessly use your own put-downs (zingers), while encouraging your real health-conscious friends to do the same—for instance, you might try calling your next door neighbor an Arrogant Anti-Athletic Aristocrat. But this is one of the biggest risks we can think of. You have enough on your plate in getting a responsible training program in place. Nevertheless, that's what women did during the women's movement. And it worked. It got all of us to think before we said anything damaging to a woman's spirit. Health-conscious-person's liberation has to eventually follow suit. Just leave it up to those who have time and energy for the battle, okay?

You want to be seen as a person who has kept at it for a long time and now has a healthiness to be proud of. This is kind of like being seen as an everyday version of an Olympic athlete, fat free, with a spring in your step, maybe a little bicep prowess for the Ponces, and a little hourglass allure for the Ms. Ds. That's nice, and that's the way it should be. But it doesn't come overnight. You have to get there first.

Nevertheless, it will start about two years from the day you begin, assuming you stick with it, eat right, and supplement. Then you will start liking what you see in the mirror as much your Ms. D or Ponce does, assuming you're working at it, preferably together. Soon after, others will notice and give you respect, thereby putting you into a class that's all your own.

But prior to that point, you will get abused. That's when you will constantly hear:

❖ "What are you trying to prove?"
❖ "You need to slow down."
❖ "Oh, didn't know you were a Health Nut."
❖ Etc.

It's during the first two years that you really need a little help from your friends. Actually, you will need more than just a little. This country is filled with the AAAA, and everyone you know is probably like this. If that weren't the case, health care would be far less expensive, and downtown, free of its current hoard of fat pedestrians, would be far more beautiful. That's why you should get close to others who are in the same place as you and get far away from your critics.

Unfortunately, the old adage, "Make new friends but keep the old," makes this very difficult. You think that you have to hang on to the old ones who have sent you Christmas cards for so many years, even when they keep putting you down. But you don't; you really don't.

If you are thinking none of this is really as bad as Ponce is making out, I will tell you that it's worse! It's physically hard starting out, and those on whom you rely emotionally do not want you to make it. Not only will you have sore muscles to start, but you will also have emotional discomfort (feeling one down) from their comments, the longer you stay at it. You will be told over and over again that you're a Health Nut.

Of course, the Normal Majority says that it's for your highest well-being that they are the way they are. Being a Health Nut following your high school mania, is sure to getcha in the end, so we'll help by getting you off the hook. They're only thinking of you, you see. After all, that's what real friends are for, right?

Friends, drop these folks along with the Mountain Dew and McDonald's. *All* of them are really bad for you.

Conclusion

Do risk being called a Health Nut.
Don't ever take it seriously.

9

Your Morning Cigarette, Coffee, and Donut

A long time ago Jack LaLanne made a point about morning breakfasts. He asked if you would ever mix up a donut, a cigarette, and a cup of coffee in a blender and give it to your pet. Everyone was horrified. Yet that is what a lot of people were doing to themselves back then. Of course, that was his point

If you remember back to the 1960s and even into the 1970s, people were starting the day off with that cigarette, cup of coffee, and donut. That was an okay thing to do even for homemakers around children. There was no concern about secondhand smoke, which they didn't know much about back then. I expect that many are still doing it today, though Ms. D and I really don't know of anyone who does. The smoking ban has actually worked, making the number of smokers far fewer today than ten years ago. But the coffee and donuts folks are still out there.

So maybe we should ask how many still dare to share their coffee and donuts with their faithful dog. But we'd rather you did the asking. That's the easiest way for you to see our point and for us to keep out of harm's way. What you will find is that people won't share the bad stuff with their pets, even though they will have no trouble ingesting it themselves. Furthermore, they will think you are odd for asking. According to them, the Normal Majority, everyone ought to know that people food is for people and dog food is for dogs.

The mature grown-up's illusion about himself is that he is built to last forever (even though he loves to talk about death and taxes). That makes him more durable than a standard poodle and, in his mind, more reliable than his Health Nut neighbor, who wouldn't dream of missing his morning run, protein shake, and supplement pack. Any such strange person, disinclined to act his age, ought to know that a lifestyle of this intensity will make him fall apart prematurely. But Health Nuts don't see it this way and must therefore learn the hard way. That makes them fair game for jokes and no sympathy when they pull a muscle. It's not quite as bad for the Ms. Ds, but they get their share of problematic glances from their suspicious lady friends.

Without that morning donut, coffee, and maybe a Camel, people might just get right into their daily routines. They might, even if they didn't want to. Most, of course, do not want to, and therefore don't do it straight away; that is something for which we can't really blame them. The average job is anything but vital, invoking no one's passion other than the CEO's at the top with his or her bonus. Even though these folks should throw themselves into the day, hoping it will get better as it goes on, they don't. Instead they do the coffee and donuts ritual. That's because saying no to cigarettes, coffee, donuts, and some laughs with your friends is rather bland, to say nothing of dangerous.

Being this way can get you labeled as a snob, introvert, or outright people-hater. In other words, not being into the coffin nails, white sugar, and thirty-two-ounce cuppa can make the normal folks wonder whether you care about life at all. So if you're not like this, you can see why they want to save you, right?

Furthermore, just because the Health Nuts look good today, there is no guarantee that they'll look just as good tomorrow. That's how the Normal Majority's litany drones on at every sad opportunity. We're always reminded that cumulative wearout or injuries hang over the heads of the athletic achievers. It's not at all like being a laid-back couch potato, a normal person, a good Joe, a nice guy, a nice gal, or a Betty (instead of Elizabeth). Being like that pretty much guarantees that you'll never slip into any of the ills of not acting your age. Granted, you may not look great, but at least in your sixties you'll still be laughing at those who have worn out or gotten injured as a result of athletics in their fifties.

Really believing those sports are gonna getcha is supposed to make it okay for the couch potatoes to not work out. Not doing so is what they expect will keep them from becoming gym rats, more aggressive and unacceptable variations of Health Nuts. That's because working out to be healthy is only mildly problematic and probably not harmful (although there's no real proof that it's any help, so their Harvard report from twenty-five years ago says), but actually trying to beat your opponent on the handball court or win the marathon is completely off the charts.

According to the Normal Majority, having such aspirations to win is okay when you're young, maybe, but not when you're our age. Other things are supposed to be far more important, like taking it easy with your friends and not doing anything to disrupt the peace. We're all in this together, remember?

That's why you as a Health Nut need to occasionally have a donut and coffee, put yourself down by talking about your knee injury from running around the block in the morning like you shouldn't, and offer to pay for breakfast. Yes, I am being facetious, but these will buy you some time if things get tense, as they almost always will. They will get you off the firing line, forcing the normal people to find some others who are more troubling to focus on, such as those who insist on buying SUVs instead of pickups.

You actually might keep this option in the back of your mind for purposes of self-preservation. You can always make a joke about yourself and/or pay for everyone else's poison, including your own. That will work, as what's really going on is their discomfort at your success, which you are purposely causing.

Your friends, Fred and Bart, are getting envious (rather, you're making them feel that way) of your resolve to run every morning, largely because it makes you look thinner. That's why you owe them. You are purposely disrupting their peace. By putting yourself down and eating some of those donuts with that big cup of coffee, you can come across as an okay person again, or at least as someone who's trying to make things right. Sounds like exactly what you should do, doesn't it?

Everyone should want to be sensibly healthy, but underline the word *sensibly*. Anything more makes the Normal Majority uptight. Therefore, you shouldn't want to be anything more. So if you are a Dara Torres type wanting the equivalent of another Olympic gold at forty-six, you have got to either give it up or keep quiet about her, since no one can really understand her. And you, well, you're out there training like she is. How is that possible? Don't you both have kids?

Being consistent and disciplined really makes both you and Dara suspect. But it gets worse. Trust me, when your athletic lifestyle starts paying off, when you start getting really good, they'll wonder if you're on steroids. The only reason Dara escaped this suspicion is because of her appearance (doesn't look or sound mannish—kinda pretty, in fact). Luckily, attention turned from her victories to the country's new president, Obama, so scrutiny of her never got out of hand. When you, on the other hand, start getting really good, you may not be so lucky even if there's a lot going on politically.

In other words, to the Normal Majority, normal is okay, but beyond that it is iffy, largely because they think it's not humanly possible. So when you start getting up to a daily ten-miler, you will be pretty close to being as badly off as Dara with a gold medal at forty-two. (Two to three miles of everyday laps in a fifty-meter pool are not even remotely comprehensible.) Doing that kind of thing makes the Normal Majority come unglued! For sure, so they think, it must be dangerous, something which *will*, not *may*, result in injury or wearout in the not too distant future.

Assuming the Normal Majority has seen something before, it's probably safe. At least that's what they believe, and this is what everyone believes, right? So swimming a few laps now and then is probably safe. They've seen it or can imagine it. But swimming two miles before breakfast is something different. They've never seen it and can't possibly imagine it. The same goes for a power boost formula in a can after an hour swim followed later on by weight training. That's a little strange or a little different, as they say in Minnesota.

That's why you seldom see or hear of people doing anything so Torres-like. It may be happening, but no one in their right mind is going to let the Normal Majority know what they're up to. People living in a health-conscious way (doing maybe only one mile in a twenty-five-yard pool, seventy-two daily laps—nothing too shabby, by the way), who can't get away from the Normal Majority, have to keep a low profile and let everyone else choose the topics of conversation.

People like Dara are not normal and they really do not appear to be the worse for it. That's the real problem. If only they looked haggard for all their extra work and reduced calories! But they don't. Therefore, they screw up the standard expectations and beliefs of the Normal Majority. The fact is that athletic people all look younger, lighter, more hopeful, and with it. In other words, they de-age, which is what everybody wants, right? So how can they possibly be in a nearly nonexistent minority?

The standard answer has been that it's physically hard to be a champion at any age, especially so after forty. The body supposedly slows down every year after birth until there is nothing left. Maybe it does, assuming our superstars LaLanne and Torres are fundamentally, perhaps genetically, different from the Normal Majority. In other words, the Normal Majority may be right in thinking that these people are freaks of nature.

Okay ... maybe. But how much do we ourselves bring about our wrinkles, aches, and pains by not having the courage to swim outside the box (keep up the workouts after forty)? And how much is due to that daily coffee-and-donut routine, to say nothing of what it's followed by with the other real meals (not from the organic market) for lunch and dinner seven days a week and fifty-two weeks a year. This is not a test. (Just kidding!)

When you compare the appearance of Dara to other forty-two-year-olds, or any older athlete, it's rather bewildering. Just on the basis of her example, how can there not be many other fit, happy forty-year-olds who wouldn't think of eating donuts, drinking too much coffee, or missing a workout? After all, Dara is like this, so why not them? Surely everyone knows that she would never stoop to that, don't they? Wouldn't you think that there would be thousands of Dara devotees, something like groupies around Madonna?

You might think there should be, but, unfortunately, that just isn't the way it is. If it were, you'd have a far easier time of it. So why are things the way they are?

Ms. D and I think that it's because of the extraordinarily effective advertising media, which lulls the country into thinking that the good life with its "take it easy"s and "have a great day"s is as good as it gets. Furthermore, the FDA-approved American fun food (from M&Ms to Mac and Dons, IHOP to Arby's) is not only attractive, but believed to be the best of all possible worlds for us. There are even some who believe these are superior to organic food, for reasons that aren't even remotely clear. (It tastes good, as if the co-op organic food doesn't, and apparently sticks to your ribs.) Put that together with the opinions from your next door neighbor and the advice of your MD and you have an unparalleled intellectual tour de force: a mass brainwashing of the American public.

As a team, they can make everyone think of nothing other than grabbing a burger and fries after mowing the grass on Saturday. Same goes for donuts and coffee. (Luckily, cigarettes are now considered addictive, which wasn't the case fifteen years ago.) These folks even have the power to make you think that taking Sunday to rest up by doing nothing other than walking from the car into church is the very thing that you need every week, even when it follows a sedentary Saturday.

Doing a workout falls into the same manner of thinking. Exercise—meaning five to ten chin-ups, five to six blocks of walking, and a little golf—is okay, but intense daily weight training, e.g.. a daily five to ten miles of running plus a weekend of rock climbing on Saturday and Sunday just for diversion, is a bit extreme. Too much intensity turns you into a freak: an *extreme* Health Nut, right?

Of course it doesn't, but we'd rather not enlighten your critics for you. After all, it's easier on us if you just put yourself down and buy everyone donuts and coffee, isn't it? Sorry.

In a like manner, watching what you eat is okay, if this means having no more than two and a half cheeseburgers a week with maybe a beer or two in between those real meals with the meat and potatoes. But eating like a champion is presumably asking for trouble. In other words, eating low-fat, low-carb foods along with lots of fruits and veggies every day (not the kind of food that gives you diarrhea) is courting missed appointments and having your stomach growl before the next meal. How unseemly—oh my! Too much healthy austerity isn't good for you, right? Better are those daily morning coffee and donut sit-downs with your Normal Majority coworker friends, followed by a good lunch, wouldn't you agree?

Friends, if you want to look like almost everyone on the street, then eat and exercise like most everyone on the street. That's the most certain way of pulling this off. Then everyone will think you are a good person, somebody just like them. Always aspire to this mediocrity and you'll remain safe. It may even make your friends pay for the coffee and donuts more than half the time.

Do what you want. As soon as someone more questionable comes up, you'll be off the hook. All we ask is that you never make an announcement saying you want to look like a Bowflex model or that you don't care that Jack LaLanne wore jumpsuits. These will really get you into trouble.

Just always remember that athletic excellence is wonderful for heroes in magazines or the jet set, but not for normal people. Forget about what it can do for your health. Everyone is supposed to know that regular intense workouts are gonna getcha sooner than later if you're over thirty-five. Sharing in everyone's beliefs will keep you safe and get you invited to the coffee and donut shop every morning. What could possibly be more desirable?

That is why Ms. D and I change the subject when talk turns to people like Dara at forty-two or LaLanne at ninety-five. This, of course, assumes we couldn't get out of having to be with the people talking in the first place. Dara and LaLanne are living examples of what anyone can do with their bodies if they just keep working at them. The trouble is that no one else seems to see it that way.

Of course, there are growing numbers of very healthy people, although they are not as prominent as LaLanne or Torres. They're out there, and you might even know them. Sometimes they're talked of as fifty-one going on thirty-three, and the like. Some may not have even gone out for sports in high school, but they are late bloomers in exceptional condition, largely due to their own efforts. Maybe one or two of these even go to your place of worship. They are the ones with the trim waistlines and the spring in their step. Take them out for tofu and herbal tea! They should be your friends if for no reason other than they will never do the coffee and donut shuffle.

The question is: "How do you relate to these quasi-superstars?" If they go to your church, are they good Christian folk just like yourself? Or do you see them as freaks, possibly the odd result of a rare gene or two? Or are they in need of a psychiatrist, unable to keep from doing things that suggest an inability to accept their actual ages? Or maybe they're just a little different … people you should make sure your kids don't get too friendly with. Possibly, you won't even greet these unusual persons unless you absolutely have to. (Hopefully that's not the case, but it might be, at least for right now.)

This is the primary reason that so many look as couch potato-ish as they do. They think the in-shape people are strange, unlike the coffee, cigarette, and donut real people, and aren't capable of mainstream living. And having your kids take after them would be the epitome of bad parenting, wouldn't it? Please—stop the music.

Ms. D and I think you should make friends with at least one of these seemingly from-Neptune individuals. Talk with the person and see if he or she is really as bad as the Normal Majority believes. That's what you'll have to do if you want to change yourself. You're simply going to have to be deeply convinced that your basic humanity will not be jeopardized by becoming exceptional. The best way to do that is to actually befriend one of them. Of course, it will also help to drop the morning coffee and donuts routine along with all of the excuses for not working out, but we know you've been working on these since the start of the year, right?

We all know what we have to do to look the way we want. But we don't do it. Hanging on to the coffee and donut real people is one of the big reasons. Giving these up for a never-ending Lent is a great place to start. Replacing them with some awesome others is an even better one.

Conclusion

Do treat yourself as well as you treat your pets.
Don't be afraid to make a new health-conscious friend.

10

A Little Help from Your (Real) Friends

Yes, we're just like you. We think that facts should be presented coolly and that people ought to make up their own minds about what to do with them. We are sure that you would agree strongly with us. But when it comes to the W word (for workout), I'm not sure that it's in anyone's best interest to be so reasonable. For instance, you wouldn't say: "On the basis of the following studies it has been shown that—yada yada yada—it's probably best if you consider exercise in moderation, don't you think?"

We doubt it. You'd think that your friends ought to just dive into working out with no excuses, right? That's what you'd advise your best friend, wouldn't you? Or would you still say, "That really sounds like a pretty big risk, considering how bad off you look, so you should really see what your doctor has to say"? Would you really say this to anyone? Sure, you may know of some whom you should say that to, but how many of them are there, really?

The same goes for diet and supplementation, but these never pose as much of a problem. You know that you can always say "Just eat less and exercise more" without raising too many eyebrows. People know they have to do something other than all of the normal stuff that gets no one anywhere. For all practical purposes, they know that eating like a pig will make you look like one, so there really isn't much that needs to be said about eating right.

Nevertheless, for some who come from families where you have to eat certain foods (so mom won't feel bad), this is still a big deal. These are generally the same families that get fat trying to prove that three square meals in addition to TGIF and TGIS malts, cheeseburgers, fries, and a few beers now and then along with a chocolate sundae or two (just for a weekend reward, of course) are all you need for health and energy as long as you don't smoke (much).

The long and short of it is that some folks just don't get it, and these may be the very same folks who are important to you. You may still be friends with some people like this, in spite of us telling you to drop them. So you have to be very careful. We cannot emphasize this enough. It's either that or you have to stay away from them completely. We know that's probably impossible, at least when you're a newbie.

Our guess is that you already know this and only need a little help from us to make it easier to stay away from the temptation to go back to the old ways. You have to remember that your old friends have the power to pull you back, to make you say yes when you should say no and vice versa. That's pretty normal, as none of this is easy until you've been at it for a couple of years.

Even then, it can still be tough, especially when you are around people you care about. It's sometimes even hard around those you don't care about, like strangers waiting to board a plane. They can become problematic when seen reveling in their Coney Islands, Cokes, and ice cream. (Here we're talking a relatively fibreless 1,000-plus-calorie snack with 300 to 500 calories for the soft drinks, polished off with a high fat turtle sundae of 600 calories. This feast is followed by not only hours of sitting on the plane, but probably a real food high-carb, high-fat dinner and not even a nightly stroll around the block prior to going to sleep.) Sounds like an awesome blowout, right? Maybe even a well-deserved treat, as there was an airline delay.

When confronted by a situation like this, you may get completely confused about what's right. There are some okay others, not all that much different from yourself, who seem to find it enjoyable to dig their graves with their teeth.

Fascinating, how humanly enjoyable this really appears to be! Can having that kind of fun really be all that bad?, you might ask. Here I am trying to stay the course like this Health Nut Ponce and his wife expect; plus, I've been good for a whole two weeks. Could it be that I'm being a bit too gung ho, or a bit more Spartan than is good for me?

This is particularly troubling when you suddenly remember that the Internet is a cyberlibrary of facts, theories, workout routines, supplements, diets, and exercises for the exercise-hater, and that you have heavily bought into it. You probably get e-mails about our favorite fountains of youth like resveratrol or acai berries, and you may even have a few websites in your favorites folder, feeding you all sorts of diet and supplement advice. The same goes for advice on workouts.

In other words, you've done your homework. You're part of today's healthiness, so it seems. But here you are in the airport sitting across from folks who are just having a good time—the same type your buddies back home are into, possibly every weekend. Can it be that so many others aren't as much into being health conscious as you, or worse, that they don't even seem to care? What does this say about you as a human being?

Watch out. The Normal Majority is gaining on you. A newbie has that to look forward to. And that is the point of this chapter. (Pssst. That's why you need some new friends, badly, and right now. Where's your cell phone? You do have Iron Man Ed's number programmed in, don't you?)

How can the Normal Majority still be so influential as to make you feel like a complete nut instead of just a Health Nut?, you wonder. We're not completely sure, but Ms. D and I think it's because the media has done such overkill on the safe and fun aspects of the American good life that people still find it almost impossible to live any differently. So you are not alone. The old tried and true is tried and supposedly the only true. It's normal. It's the way to be. It's American. It's easy, fun, attractive, appealing, and right there for you to enjoy.

That's why people who want to get off the sauce of normality—you—really need a little (a whole lot of) help from your (new) friends: people who, like you, are already committed to working out, dieting, and supplementing. You may agree to that but wonder why you still feel so much like you are going to slide backward.

The standard answer to this question has always been that most people do not really want to be any different. In other words, they just *say* they do. It's almost as if they're being phony about their aspirations. This has been the primary psychological answer to people who wonder why they can't stay on a diet or stick with working out. We disagree.

We believe that lots of people fundamentally really do, *yes, really do*, want to change but find that they are continually tempted to go back to the old ways. This is particularly upsetting to them, and many times results in missed workouts or blown diets. How can that be when they—very good, responsible and mature adults—know it shouldn't be?

Our belief is that there are parts of them that want to stay the same. The people may not be all that aware of them, but those parts are there and they're very strong. They remain powerful for a very long time, let's say for two to three years, until you start seeing very significant changes that make you say, "I'm no longer the 'me' that I once was, and the mirror agrees." Then this becomes less trouble. But we're talking two to three years down the road, not this afternoon! (Freud said these thoughts never really go away.) So try as a person will, he or she has to do a lot to really make it. And much of that can really be quite confusing, to say nothing of scary.

For instance, you would think that looking like a swimsuit model would be something everybody craves. They do, to be sure. But, the newfound attractiveness of being forty pounds lighter often times causes acute anxiety. The mere presence of that new image, long before the exertion of any effort at all, will do the dastardly trick. Besides: "How many others at my age aren't doing anything like what I'm up to?" That's how great plans never get followed through on.

Becoming dramatically trimmer raises scary questions in those who were not this way before. Questions come up such as: "Who will expect what of me now when I am so attractive?" and "What doors will this open up that I am not prepared to walk through?"

Fat not only holds you back because of its sheer weight, making it too hard in most cases to run a nightly five miles (or do thirty minutes on a NordicTrack, if five miles on the street sounds like from here to the North Pole), but it also protects you from other opportunities for which you may not be in the least prepared. Being a candidate for them now changes everything.

That's why a considerable number of people read the helpful tips on how to lose those love handles by July but never once set foot in a gym. Or they change their ways for a few weeks, only to go back to the same old habits. Doing so ensures that they will look like the same old Joe/Joanne they always were, which will allow them to keep fitting right in with all of their couch potato friends. And yes, there's way more of them than there are aspiring health-conscious persons, just like you.

The same goes for reading about how to cut fat or carbs while continuing to frequent Mac and Dons for the weekly TGIF celebration. As long as you are starting on Monday to get psyched up for the weekly Friday real food blowout, it is unlikely that you will be doing any real Health Nut fat and carb cutting for the rest of the week. That little cheating during the week will keep you popular.

Everybody wants to fit in and be like everyone else. Granted, everyone also wants to feel unique, but the feeling of being normal is most important. It's primary. This feeling comes chiefly from how others see us. If they like what they see, we feel we're okay. If not, we don't, and when it comes to a person's appearance this is especially so. Your friends have to approve of it as okay. If it's thought that you're on the way to becoming a Bowflex model, it won't be okay. The same goes for becoming obese, on the flip side.

The sure way to keep your peers happy is to stay pretty much the way you are. But pretty much the same is not exactly the same, which is okay, and the Normal Majority will cut you some slack. A little deviation is only to be expected, as no one is a machine. For example, a little "puttin' it on lately" is okay as long as there's one of Oprah's diet secrets in your near future. But really porking out (becoming obese), with none of Oprah's berry juice (acai) in the offing, is not. Similarly, being a little too pooped to participate (especially if after a well-deserved weekend blowout) is okay, whereas becoming sedentary and almost always refusing an invitation for a weekend golf game is asking for trouble.

So much for the grace from your almighty peer group. Announcing that you are going to become an athlete is crossing the line into sin. Our advice is to keep your mouth shut about such blatant deviance (or is it sinfulness), but you may not like our underhanded approach. Okay, do what you must, but remember, becoming an athlete is seen as becoming someone you're not. Forget about whether you'll actually be able to do so only after a relatively long period. It's the intent that does it; besides, you might have some secret something about you that could make the difference. That's why six months instead of thirty-six worth of regular full miles in the pool just might transform you into Michael Phelps or Dara Torres. Stranger things have happened. *They* oughta know.

As long as there is a perceived way back to the same old you, and you're humble enough to listen, no one will care much about what you do. The Normal Majority can always encourage you with a "Liked you better when you weren't so gung ho." This, they believe, will always work and, sadly, they are generally dead correct. They want you to return to the golden age of being like everyone else, which means acting your age.

In other words, they like you best when *they* are still in control. Consequently, there will never be a problem unless you give the impression that you are going after a personal transformation in spite of them. Becoming a whole other person is never okay unless they give you permission, which they never will. The easy way to say this is that your clothes can fit a little more loosely, but you can never find it necessary to buy a whole new wardrobe.

That's what you go through in the real world with people you've been conditioned to call your friends (your old ones). And it's the chief reason you don't stick with the routine you start out with to make the changes you deserve. For lack of a better way to say it, you want to remain loyal and you know that you owe them (or, as we would say it, we know you *think* you do). That will make you hang on to the old habits that you absolutely must give up.

What you need are some new friends to help you break away from the old ones. Those are people who will get excited about your changes, possibly because they're going through the same thing. No matter how independent you believe you are, you need their help. You cannot make it alone. Without some new people to pull you up, you will simply be subject to the old ones, who will pull you down. That's the way we all are—social animals in need of being like others. The faster you realize this, the faster you'll start transforming.

The personal, or internal, side of the problem is a little different. This is what you experience inside yourself with the imaginary people who live inside your head, so to speak. It's what you go through alone or with a psychologist. Therefore, it's something you really can't share with the Normal Majority folks who are closest to you. They don't ever like conversations that include "If you're hearin' voices inside your head, you must be crazy." But it's something you have to deal with, just as you would with real, everyday people. The imaginary people are there with you when you are alone, and they're equally, if not even more, perturbing. Ignoring them won't make them go away.

To illustrate, let's assume that you erroneously take to heart what you've been promised by a fitness guru. In under a month of starting a weight training routine, possibly on a Bowflex or something similar, you will transform into a mid-forties version of a *Baywatch* lookalike, so he has assured you. That's what you've been promised. Maybe you've seen him on YouTube; that makes him even *more* for real. Whatever the case, this person is now part of your imagination, promising you overnight miracles. You, being a bit gullible and the proud owner of a brand new piece of gym equipment, believe him, and he is alive in your imagination. That's the good news.

The bad is that very soon you are going to have to act a new part in the real world. That's what you believe, at least. It means that you will need to come up with lines you've never rehearsed and deal with folks you never met. Mentally, you may even start gravitating toward a more prestigious area or suburb where the better-off people do things that you've never even thought about. They may all sound exciting, but they may just be too frightening if you realize that you will actually have to do them. Besides, you can't afford a new mortgage.

Those fears can be enough to make you quit before you even get started. In other words, it's not so much that the new machine doesn't work, but that you suddenly find reasons for not even using it. You have been defeated before you even start.

Instead of going through the necessary changes and adaptations (realistically doing so over at least six months), you choose to forgo all of the physical training on the front end. Thus, you simply nip it all in the bud, thinking of the time and maybe money you'll save. Besides, it's far less stressful to just be your normal self—even if being in shape might forever cure you of high blood pressure and heart disease! That's the mature thing to do at your age anyway, isn't it? So why not just leave the kid stuff of being someone you're not to the Health Nuts? Then your life will stay intact, making it far easier to do the things that are expected of you. This is another way of acting your age, or being mature.

Ms. D's and my answer to this sad thinking is that transformations don't happen overnight and people need friends who will stand with them as they go through the agony. People need real friends—ones who can share an occasional "I've been there too" or "Give yourself some time." People need real friends to help them take stands against the people in their heads and the real ones at church. We all need someone on our side, someone going through what we're going through, preferably someone who's made it past the impasses. That's a whole different person from a mature, stodgy adult in the Normal Majority who knows that if only you had been acting your age, you never would have wasted your time or money on anything that high school–like in the first place.

Once you have the right people to talk with, you can get them into your imagination as well. That comes in handy if they're not around to pick up the phone when you need them. The same goes for you in relation to other folks. When the

Normal Majority starts getting you down (again), you can just think about your friends in other states, one of whom might just have won the marathon at age forty-six. Talk about a great use of the Internet and the ultimate upper in the face of the blahs!

You need this desperately. It's the only way to live among the Normal Majority without being held back by them. It's also the only way to keep up your spirits when the second month of never missing your Bowflex routine, or the full mile swim in the pool, doesn't seem to working out for you. This is the time when you have to hear "Hang in there. It'll do what you want, but it's going to be on *its* time schedule." That will keep you doing what you need to be doing so that everything you're doing can do its thing.

There has to be someone in your life in whom you can confide. Of course, that should be either your Ponce or MsD, but having a few more who say the same good things is always a blessing. One can never have enough good friends. There is strength in numbers and what you need to remember is that the world is primarily all Normal Majority. They're everywhere and even have friends in high places, so they're proud to report (presumably such as the AMA and the doctors).

Perhaps you are thinking that it will wreck everything with all of your old friends if you are silly enough to listen to us. More than likely, it will. To be honest, we do think you'll be better off without them, though alienating them is dangerous. That's why we think you need to keep a stiff upper lip while you make new friends. The Internet is good for that, as you can start your own support group (or join ours). All you really need to do is be honest. Just type in, "workout friends" and be willing to say, "I need some new people to grow with, as all of my lifelong friends can't help but hold me back. So if you've just started up a training program and need someone to talk to …" This should help you find real friends who share your love for living forever, enabling you to keep on getting healthier.

The point is that being told by a friend to keep it up offers the best chance of getting you to the gym tomorrow. This is the opposite of "Better take it easy" or "You're not as young as you used to be." The encouragement gives you a boost without your having the slightest idea why; the caution dampens your spirits and maybe even causes extreme self-doubt. That's because of what's being said by whom. Words from others simply have a very powerful effect on you. Do not think you are above this; you aren't. Words really have an affect at a subliminal level. In other words, you don't even realize that someone's words got you over to gym until after you actually get there. Or did the words you heard make you think that maybe you should just take today off after all of your hard work last week?

It doesn't stop with verbal communication. Being ignored or even being given an indirect message of envy can have negative effect as well. (This is the opposite of "Send me a pic today and another in a month.") When no one seems to care about how you look or what you do, you start to lose confidence. You may say, "They're just being that way to me because they're jealous." Or you may doubt the reality of the very good changes you are starting to see in the mirror. That's okay. It's just that you don't want to be saying, "Maybe the three fewer inches on my waistline one only in my imagination!" The long and short of it is that people who play indifferent to you will not have the same positive effect on you as a real friend who asks for before-and-after photos. Nevertheless, they will have an effect. Therefore your old friends should be avoided, assuming you can do that. (But we know that, realistically, you may not be able to for some time.)

Ms. D and I think that everyone just starting out will need a new group of friends to encourage them. Taking it easy, going to Mac and Dons, and thinking you just pee vitamins away anyway are too much a part of American life. Too many people are still saying things like this, making you feel weird for not playing along. The Normal Majority is still about all of this and that is the bulk of the problem. Sadly, they are almost always the ones who are the closest to you and most influential over you. That's why you need some new friends, so that you just won't have as much (or any) time for the old ones.

The bottom line is simple: to change your body you need to first change your circle of friends. If you don't, you will indefinitely put off buying the vitamins, the low-fat, low-carb groceries, and the health club membership. Or you will find your new bottle of multivitamins one-third full two months from now, and make one excuse after another for not doing your workouts. The effects of people on people are subtle, but they're strong. They can result in your inconsistency or your great success. Your success has a lot to do with you, to be sure, but it's about others as well. You absolutely have to accept this fact.

Conclusion

Do find a support group.
Don't let your lifelong friends shorten your life span.

11

If Okay Isn't Good Enough, You Need DeLeonitor

The title of this chapter is a spoof on the latest ads that say that if diet and exercise aren't enough, you need this month's wonder of modern science—a brand new pill. What we believe is that if diet and exercise aren't enough, you haven't been doing them long enough or hard enough. So DeLeonitor is nothing more than GOFHW: good old fashioned hard work.

Being that direct in a permissive decade puts us into the harsh or rude category. But we really don't care. Someone has got to put his foot down, ending the fast-food, fast-cure, fast-fix, fast-makeover country we live in. That's why we're recommending DeLeonitor as an answer to your aging right on schedule, or your unfortunate lack of shapeliness, if that sounds better.

DeLeonitor is us and what we have to say. That's everything having to do with systematic, diligent, disciplined diet, exercise, and supplementation. Overdoses of it will have no side effects (with the possible exception of a little muscle soreness), and no prescription is necessary. You needn't even ask your MD first, unless you just can't hold yourself back. In fact, we'd rather you just surprised him or her with the results after six months of our wonder drug.

Of course, you can prove us to be charlatans if you underdo or overdo. But we are counting on you to use your head. That is the big difference between us and the doctor promoters. We think you still have the brain God gave you. On the other hand, the Normal Majority thinks the doctors know more about you than you do (which would seem remarkable, as your MD sees you for only about twenty minutes twice a year).

But just in case you are radically unsure of yourself, you are probably wondering whether you should first ask your MD if we're okay. So here's our question in answer to your question: "Would you ask your MD if you were healthy enough for sex?" If your answer is yes, then don't read this book; give it to one of your friends. That is the ultimate as far as we're concerned, and there really was a commercial that suggested doing just that. If you have to ask if you're healthy enough for the "big s," you'll have to ask about the big GOFHW as well.

Friends, you should know who you can trust, but you might not. Even though we are in better shape than your younger physician, some of you will still prefer what he or she has to say even about fitness, which is really not his or her expertise. Chalk it up to media influences, presumably. The Normal Majority says don't do anything until you check with your MD first, so that's what you'll have to do.

But we'd really love it if you tried to get over that. Why would you go to a $15 per hour personal banker when you need investment advice? A $200 K per year stock broker would make more sense, wouldn't it? I know that's cruel, but that is the way it is. MDs make you better when you're sick, or they mend bones when they get broken. That's what they do in addition to some very complex operations. That's a lot, but that's it. Do not expect them to show you the way to beach readiness.

Most of us go to the MD to either get healthy or stay healthy. That is, you go when you're sick or you go to get a checkup. That's pretty normal. It is like going to the bank to make a withdrawal or a deposit, assuming you have an income. Everybody does this from time to time. But, just like some of us, if you dream about Powerball types of things (such as looking like a fitness magazine foldout), doing only the normal thing just might not be enough. That's particularly true when it comes to health.

If you are in this category, if you'd like to look like Jane Fonda or Sly Stallone, you will be frustrated by the help you cannot get from your doctor. It's just like what you will never get from your bank when it comes to an amazing opportunity. (They think there isn't anything as amazing as their regular paycheck. That's why it's tough, if not impossible, to get venture capital.) In other words, expecting advice about how to look good on the beach is like asking the bank for help in making stock purchases. Bankers don't get into that type of thing.

Some of us dare to look good on the beach. Yes, I used the word "dare." It takes courage to say that you want to look good on the beach (at fifty and up), and my guess is that it even does for twenty-year-olds. There are a vast number of young people who look as bad as their parents and grandparents do. Lately, the TV has been blaming it on sugar-loaded soda consumption (e.g., Mountain Dew), but there are other reasons for being so unfit. These have chiefly to do with not working out. Kids are also unable to do this. Our guess is that they are getting called Health Nut every time they say that they want to achieve anything from a respected place on the high school swimming team to a coveted one on the USA Olympic team. "Who do ya think you are, Michael Phelps?" may be what they're getting every morning with their milk and cereal (if they even get that).

As I write this, I am wondering who is going to think less of us Health Nuts for being so vain or immature. After all, Ms. D and I are well over the age of forty and I keep saying the best motivator for being forever fit is staying in shape to look good on the beach. How immature can you get?

Of course, that's only a means to the great end of being fat free, energetic, and positive, but what Normal Majority fanatic would ever believe that? We're just Health Nuts and there are no two ways about it. The only thing that's worse is that the next person I see on the street will actually call his own son or daughter a Health Nut, saying, "Spendin' time playin' at sports instead of doin' you homework and bein' a regular kid, ain'tcha?"

As far as high school per se is concerned, we think that any homework routine will be greatly enhanced by a workout routine. Our critics, the Normal Majority, just can't get up to speed when it comes to that. They're supposedly so high-minded (moral or something), caring only for the overall good of society. Perhaps they are, but I refuse to say that they're really all that well intentioned. Possibly they were out for a sport in high school and mom watched their grades suffer, but we doubt it. We just know of far too many stories that are the opposite. Further, studies in the 1960s proved that athletics are helpful. That's why we think that kids as well adults ought to be on DeLeoniter. It might even make them look better on the beach, while they still have those wild oats to sow. (Or is that too problematically vain for the Normal Majority?)

Only the Health Nuts would care about looking good on the beach. That's what the Normal Majority believes. For them, sensible people care only about being healthy enough to make it to the beach, possibly walking there if it's not more than a couple of miles. That's the type of exertion that's adequate for anyone. Those who want more are suspected of being in their second adolescence. Where can this wisdom be coming from?

It's true that those who look good are doing the right things on a daily basis. This takes a lot of work and intense dedication, at least in the beginning. (It gets way easier, believe me.) Those are super-adult habits, a far cry from being immature. Surely everyone would agree, wouldn't they? So how then can it be that people get called Health Nuts for being so dedicated (or compulsive, as their critics say)?

Ms. D and I would agree that there is nothing wrong with being ten or fifteen pounds overweight, having a few sags, always feeling tired and worn out—if that's what you really want for yourself. But do you? Is that really what you want for you? Granted, there are no laws against it, and some people think it makes you come across as being real.

Looking dowdy and feeling overburdened makes you look serious and important. Furthermore, it hurts no one, unless you are thinking about your spouse, who is stuck with you for life. (Actually, we have a certain amount of indignation over this, but married couch potatoes tend to be comfortable with their hubbies and wifeys the way they are.) There is no actual law against looking like a couch potato. Maybe that is one of the reasons that there are so many?

Of course, there are the unwritten laws against being a couch potato. And these can keep you from being promoted or even hired in the first place. But those things don't really count, so we're taught to believe. They're only there to allow one to get angry at superficial folks like Ms. D and me, apparently, who seem to base so much on appearance. Or is it that we just want to get our two Mercedes by getting everyone on DeLeonitor?

The Normal Majority believes that one's body is not something to be criticized unless it falls into the category of obesity or anorexia. As long as you're not either of these, you're okay. What's really important is just all-around good health, whatever that really means. Most of the time we think it suggests having passed your physical when you see the doctor. He or she is the grand and glorious person who bestows the okay blessing, right? Our question is simply this: "Is that okay stamp from this important person good enough for you and for your MsD, or do you want something more?"

What most folks think is okay or healthy is not something that Ms. D and I ever wanted for either of us. That means we never wanted to be pleasantly dowdy. Sure, dowdy is okay, better than obese, or disease ridden like some of those poor folks in Africa. Besides, a lot of our best acquaintances still are this way. It may even look somewhat grandparent-y, and thus be romanticized, kind of like Mr. and Mrs. Claus at Christmas. That is the way that we're supposed to look when we're over the hill, being kindly grandparents, so who is to criticize anyone for that (unless they themselves want something different or better)?

Looking standard or okay for our age is all we're supposed to be into, saith the Normal Majority. Assuming you do, you will always get the expected invitations to Thanksgiving and Christmas along with occasional requests for advice that will never be followed. Same goes for all other parents and grandparents alike. It will keep you politically correct and safe.

You forfeit all of these worthwhile blessings if you start looking better than the under-thirty folks who also show up for the holidays, sitting right next to you at the table. Now *there's* a great reason to not stock up on DeLeonitor, when we've got it on sale.

Ms. D and I never cared about any of this. Sure, affection from your kids is great, but you need to pull the plug on it when they start insisting you look like their friends' elders. They do this, you know. They want you to look like their friends' grandparents because that fits with having kids of their own. Whoever would want an Iron Man Grandpa or a Distance Swimmer Granny? It doesn't fit the standard expectations. Furthermore, how could they explain to their children that the old folks are better than they are at athletics? Everyone knows their parents aren't supposed to look like they did in high school. That's weird. They are now supposed to be warm and cuddly like the AARP-y folks you see on TV. That's the way all older people are, isn't it?

Ms. D and I could never figure out why we are in a minority so small that we are statistically insignificant. How can we have been among a handful of the population who always knew that if you start letting yourself go, you are virtually unable to turn back the clock. How can so many not know this or not seem to care? Perhaps we should leave the whys and wherefores to someone else and just suggest that all people take DeLeonitor.

Once again, in case you have forgotten, it's really not much different from GOFHW. That means disciplined, healthy, systematic exertion, really good, "never miss" habits—the kind you might have had in high school when you were on the champion swim team, or that you may have now when it comes to brushing your teeth (every day at the same time in the same way with all of the best brushes and toothpastes).

DeLeonitor is our advice. That will make the difference. Take it today and next year you will think, feel, and act ten years younger. Go ask the MD or some respected "friend" at church if you should, or if it's okay, and they will probably tell you to watch it (at your age). That's a nonprohibitive way of saying "don't do it." It keeps them safe and holds you back.

You know what we think, which puts us at risk from the FBI, but maybe it spurs you on. The only question is, "Who will you let win the day?"

The freedom to move and be the person you want is yours. Hold onto it and never let it go. Start today if you haven't already done so. Put that together with the right diet and supplements and you will stay trim forever. Give yourself just six months of always taking your DeLeonitor and we're sure that you will get everyone you know to do the same. That'll get us our two Mercedes, you see. But you won't mind, will you?

Conclusion

Do get into Good Old Fashioned Hard Work
Don't think that the easy answers of today are enough.

12

The Powerball of Youth

Winning at Powerball is something most prudent people would never talk about. Sure, it happens, but the chances are one in how many million? In other words, it hardly ever does, even though there are in fact recipients of the big payoffs. Somehow the players just come up with the right numbers to win.

As fluky as it may sound, something like this can happen when you work out. It hardly ever does, but it can. To a newbie, the odds may seem the same as for Powerball but they aren't.

The fitness players win more often. This can be called physical transformation out of the blue. Maybe it is like a similar phenomenon reported by physicians called spontaneous remission: the cure of a serious condition that happens almost overnight. In our context, this is like going from average to extraordinary right before everyone's eyes.

I have seen it twice, long before any wonder supplements or anything special, about thirty or forty years ago, first in the late 1960s and next in the early 1980s. Because I have seen it twice but have never met a Powerball recipient, it makes me think that a sudden physical transformation is far more likely. But I would never recommend that you hold out for that sudden transformation, at least not until you've heard me out. Such passivity is exactly *not* what everything in this book is all about.

Talking about overnight transformations (even if overnight translates into under a month) falls in the same category as talking about flukes and how to win Powerball. If you bring it up in public, it will get you labeled as a radical, which is far to the left of Health Nut. Nobody (of the Normal Majority, that is) believes this happens, and you will be considered a little different for talking seriously about it.

To see it the way the Normal Majority sees it, you have to believe that exceptional people were hatched—born with great genes that make them look like Greek statues from the get-go. That makes them okay, as they couldn't have helped it, but it's almost always only for the under-forty people.

Superstars over forty are super suspect. That's even if they're just maintainin', largely because they're supposed to be losin' (at the appearance game, that is). Therefore, they must be on steroids or sumthin'. Therefore, if they became exceptional after a seemingly short period of time at forty-two, let's say, it's likely that they got an extreme makeover a la plastic surgery or liposuction or God knows what without ever telling anyone. This they never should have done, saith the Normal Majority. In other words, they *could* help it and took it upon themselves to do it anyway. This is the epitome of not-okay-ness. We're sure you get the drift.

Our complaint is that, in the everyday speak of the Normal Majority, becoming a health magazine foldout has nothing to do with the disciplined pursuit of exceptional health. That is, it is generally believed that it had nothing to do with responsible, controlled attainment. No one ever says, "Wow, he certainly has benefited from his years of keeping at it; I wonder how he did what he did, so I can copy it." Instead, people generally think that it had to do with genes, a radical procedure, or a steroid. They never, never, ever think that it came from GOFHW or DeLeoniter (if you read the last chapter). This is true even for the overnight transformations that they witness with their own eyes but can't talk about because that would make them quite a bit more than a little different!

I have seen transformations without anything other than consistent hard work. Granted, I am not sure how there could have been such dramatic changes in such short periods, but I have seen them, and I do have a theory some decades later. The first time was in 1968 with Patty, twenty; the second was in 1982 with Jimmy, forty. In both instances the complete and nearly sudden change was unmistakable and nothing short of remarkable. Everyone we all knew at the places we worked out could see it. We literally could not believe our eyes.

My guess is that neither Patty nor Jimmy knew what caused their transformations either. Both seemed to attribute them to simply doing far more of what they were already doing. Patty started putting more into her tennis and practice-volleying more often; Jimmy started running ten miles each workday during his lunch hour, working every day at getting faster. They both thought that the increased activity did its work, but I know that they started turning into magazine material before they upped the intensity of their training. You could see the differences in both long before you realized that their routines had become more intense.

Both were at their escalated workout levels for far less than a month before the very noticeable changes became obvious. It is possible, though unlikely, that both were drinking something like Noni Juice—a fountain of youth substitute for many back then. But it seems unlikely. Had they been doing so, they would have been trying to sell it to all of us, to sell to others, who'd sell to more, etc., etc., in an obnoxious MLM (multi-level marketing) fashion. That never happened; and none of us ever thought to ask what was going right for either of them. We were all too much in awe.

I think the real reason we didn't say anything is that there wasn't anything terribly different about what Patty and Jimmy were doing or how they were living. Or, if there was, they both kept it hidden—and I seriously doubt that. I knew both of these people personally, so I'm certain they would have said something. Both would have talked about any major lifestyle changes. All we knew was that both were living normally, which meant going to the gym, eating in moderation, and taking a multivitamin (nothing fancy back then other than a Myadec). They were doing all of these things. But that in itself wasn't going to cause someone to go from okay to magazine-cover material in under thirty days. At least nobody thought so, and anyone, meaning just about everyone from back then, will tell you that as well.

So what caused it? Shouldn't these two have been studied by UCLA or someplace else on the West Coast? (An academic hot spot for megahealth, Broomfield, Colorado, home of the Oasis Corporation, may now have to be included as a place for such a study.) After all, overnight transformations should be the ultimate in quick fixes for Fast-Everything-America, right? That is, they are the ultimate, if indeed they really did happen, and if they could really be reproduced (or their secrets bottled like fountain water).

All of us have seen the faithful person who shows up at the club regularly, always watching what they eat. And all of us have seen that they don't ever seem to change. Sometimes they even get tired-looking, and every now and then they may put on a little weight. That described Patty and Jimmy for three years.

Further, like most people who care about their health, they didn't have any of the big bad habits, just a few minor ones. They maybe, and I mean *maybe*, went to McDonald's now and then (every other month or so, not once a week), splurged on cheese cake (once a month or so, not once a week). And of course they always ate right and did their workouts. In short, neither did anything extraordinary (even if you, friends, think that's far out).

Nevertheless, in one day, it seemed, something happened. Most likely it was nothing more than the cumulative result of what they had done up to this point. (That's what I believe, at least.) But it was dramatic, and they were changed permanently afterward. They turned from ho-hum gym frequenters into inspired athletes. Patty, the tennis player, began putting everything in back of the ball and Jimmy, the pretty good runner, ran his ten miles every day, acting like an Olympic hopeful. It was as if the spirit of the sport got into both.

Both Jimmy and Patty had been going through the motions for as long as I had known them, more than three years. They made it to the club, went through their daily dozens, probably because that was pretty much what they thought they had to do. But there was nothing great about either of them. Neither aspired to be excellent; neither did anything exceptional. They just kept at what they did. There really was nothing more.

That's why their sudden transformations have been almost too bizarre to even talk about for all this time—close to thirty-five years. It didn't seem that either of them really did anything to deserve the results they attained. It was as if it was given to them. That's because the effort they put into getting there was no different from the amount that everyone seemed to be putting into *their* workouts. But their never-miss, plod-along way of training resulted in their getting to a level where their whole beings took off into warp speed.

If you have ever worked at something like course work in undergrad long enough, resigning yourself to "that's as good as gets" only to find that in one day you go all-professor, you can relate. One day everything comes together and you just *know* the material. The same goes for exercise, diet, and supplementation. It has nothing to do with steroids or extreme makeovers of any kind. Nor can it be said to have anything to do with genes in the way the Normal Majority talks about them. It is just a simple accumulation of the positive aspects of doing of what you do daily, which very gradually but then very dramatically lifts you to a new level. It's as if all is only marginally possible for a while, but then sticks together, gels, and turns into something else. I really believe that what Patty and Jimmy experienced was no more than this.

If I am right, there are some things we should all take seriously. The biggest one might be that people who never have experiences like these give up way too early. That might be right around the standard ninety days, the period right after the New Years' resolutions that the health club owners know all about. It takes a much longer time for things to dramatically change: really a few years. This is much longer than most people are willing or able to wait. Too often, the temptation is to say, "My time could be better spent elsewhere. I'm not a kid anymore." This is what causes most people to simply succumb—after day forty-five! "Can't be frittering away my time like a Health Nut" or "There are more important things to get on with in my life," and "Being a Health Nut is for people in their second childhoods": that's how grown-ups talk, isn't it?

Doing workouts while supplementing and eating right is like regularly buying a Powerball ticket. Not doing so is the only certain way to never win. If you buy one every week, let's say, you know you have a chance. Actually, you'd have a far better chance for an awesome body with regular training, but that is beside the point. What is closer to it is that by buying Powerball tickets long enough and consistently enough, you maximize the chances of actually becoming a millionaire overnight. The same goes for your extreme physical transformation, except the time to achieve it is probably far less. Not a hundred thousand years at one Powerball ticket per week (or whatever the probability and statistic folks think). Rather, it's doing the right things for two years and then taking a look at yourself in the mirror. You will not only be pleased with the result, but may also wonder what you did to deserve it.

This happens, friends. Forget the "been there, done that" authorities who have supposedly really tried but haven't made it. Stay away from couch potatoes who talk like that. They are the folks who grab for the pill that promises results when diet and exercise aren't enough, assuming their doctor thinks its right for them. They even watch CNN looking for a better one that will be coming to Walgreen's pretty soon.

Granted, a pill (a wonder of modern science) may be very effective (and a very good way to get some very quick and necessary results), but the real trouble is with the diet and exercise. The tacit assumption is that diet, supplementation, and exercise never work. Friends, they do. All you have to do is stay with them long enough and do them hard enough. So get this kind of fountain of youth thinking that doesn't require the two years of never-miss-plod-along out of your head. You need to be a dedicated athlete instead, really into GOFHW, DeLeonitor, our wonder of modern humanity! Doing that is not even close to being an American quick-fix consumer.

Where are Patty and Jimmy today? I'm not sure. All I know is that they had been at athletics for as long as I had known them, and I doubt that they ever stopped training. (Once you get into it, you never want to stop. Further, you can't really understand why everybody doesn't do the same as you.)

My guess is that Patty went forward with her tennis, possibly some local matches, and Jimmy competed annually in Duluth, Minnesota, as a marathoner. Granted, I never saw either of them on an Olympic podium getting a medal, but I expect that they are still doing what they loved so much. For our purposes of being in really great shape, or forever fit, isn't that enough?

Why did they do what they did every day, like brushing their teeth? Because it made them feel good. Neither had Olympic aspirations or even really cared about being better than any of us at what they did. They were just into good feelings, (feeling good). There was not only the post-workout high afterward, but also the healthy buzz that powered them through the entire day. And both always cared about looking good—not fat, but energetic and optimistic—maybe the way they were created! That was what kept them going. Consequently, they were as awestruck as the rest of us when they completely transformed seemingly overnight.

But again, in a nutshell this time, what really caused it? What caused each to go from okay in-shape to magazine-cover material, during a time when no one used steroids, hydroxycut, andro anything, or even—dare we say it—creatine. How and what did it? Persistence. That's the real fountain of youth. All good things come to those who wait, and miracles, like luck, come to those who continuously work hard. That's what MsD and I believe, at least. Therefore, we keep telling you to get with it and stay at it so that you can be pleasantly surprised two years from now. That's it, friends; nothing more.

Conclusion

Do stick to it.
Don't give up because it's not going fast enough.

13

American Gothic

If diet and exercise aren't enough, you haven't done them long enough or well enough. This is a radical statement—something only a senior Health Nut, like an ambitious high school coach, would say. The more polite, politically correct phrase would be: "Then you need Jerpator" or some other new drug that sounds like that. But neither Ms. D nor myself have ever felt that being polite or politically correct was good for much other than avoiding arguments.

As a result, we probably come across to most as being American Gothics (somber farmers in front of their barn in overalls with a pitch fork, if you've seen the painting). But we may be even more guilty (saith the Normal Majority) of being killjoys or insufficiently touchy-feely.

The mature, grown-up, and reasonable Normal Majority people are wondering if Ms. D and I might not be trying to draw attention to ourselves by being so different. We're supposed to know that you cannot act like a tri-athlete at sixty, because thirty-three is the alleged cutoff.

Anyone who doesn't know and honor this must be at least a Health Nut or worse, FBI bait, articulate social menaces, intelligently advocating things that the AMA presumably thinks are too risky for everyone. These include, but are not limited to, megadoses of vitamins, strict low-fat, low-carb eating, and everyday athletic training for everyone from high school onward.

Political correctness assumes that you are doing no more than your daily dozens (military presses, curls, squats, etc,), possibly with some relatively light weights (thirty pounds max), cutting down on snacks (eliminating them would most surely lead to surliness) and maybe doing just a multivitamin five times per week (which shouldn't really be all that necessary if you you're getting three square meals on a daily basis). And last but not least, staying away from all of the bad habits (such as alcohol and cigarettes, not to mention the "harder" ones). But all this may not be enough to reduce cholesterol, high blood pressure, or whatever. Should that be the case, it's probably because of your Uncle Homer and/or Aunt Alice (as the commercials have all pointed out). Therefore, you need to ask your doctor if the latest wonder of modern science is right for you.

But that's not all. I forgot about the eight glasses of water (tap is okay, never daring to say that it should be filtered unless you want to upset the neighbors, who, of course, still believe that chlorine conquers all bacteriological trouble without any side effects) and eight hours of sleep a night, even if you only need six. Of course, you really should be staying away from everything stressful too. As long as you do all of these things, you can develop a problem or two (such as high blood pressure) and blame it on your genes.

Assuming you're being sensible like this, any problem you get won't be because of you. Thus you should be able to get a prescription for something that will correct it. You may even know what drug you need because you saw it on TV. How can your doctor know better? He or she can't. Yet if he or she is so audacious as to balk, you can always get a different one, in the same network, of course. All you should have to do is ask your doctor if this month's wonder of modern science is right for you. You know the drill. Only an American Gothic type would have a problem with all that, right? (Actually, your MD should as well.)

That's political correctness a la American health in a nutshell. When someone is doing all that, even if he just started last week, one can't criticize him. Rather, he is supposed to be admired for his effort and encouraged to get one of those wonder pills from Pfizer should his genes turn out to be irregular, test or no test to verify. That little pill supposedly will get him up to speed so that maybe he will even be able to ease up on whatever else he's doing, as soon as the MD says he's okay. Now doesn't that sound good?

The Normal Majority believes the new wonder of modern science will make it so you never have to do much more than show up for next doctor visit to make certain that the side effects aren't getting you and that your symptoms are actually improving. Of course, there is never a need to find the underlying problem or a suggestion to change your lifestyle in order that you might correct it. Why? Because you're okay, just like you knew for sure anyway! Only an American Gothic would think otherwise, either about himself or you.

Too, the doctor has only so many hours in the day, so many patients she can see. Besides, she knows that you aren't smart enough to be the doctor, but won't tell you so because that would create trouble and she has a tough case right after you. So, she figures you just won't do what you must to make any lasting major physical changes and leaves it at that.

If you did find out about lifestyle, it could mean getting on a regular exercise routine, getting on a whole different diet, or getting enough essential vitamins. Giving you that message would be worse than giving you the proverbial bitter pill to swallow. Anyway, it's easier on both of you if you just take your meds, rest up, and check back in a month. Besides, that will get her paid (not enough, in our judgment) for putting up with you. Now doesn't that sound like a plan?

In the meantime, of course, your sensible living should be maintained with three square meals a day from the four food groups, maybe taking a little fun time out for a McDonald's now and then, but not more than one 1.5 times a week, especially if we're talking cheeseburgers and fries. Along with those, you might want to consider a little diet soda to wash it down. The diet variety is best, in the interest of keeping you sugar free, unlike all of the obese kids in the entire US. (There's at least one teen obesity mini-documentary every month on the evening news.) And then maybe you should take a supplement—but only one, just one—possibly a Centrum for over-fifty adults, but that's if and only if you're over fifty. Possibly you don't really even need anything like this if you're only over forty? Anyway, the MD won't talk straight about any of this, so you're on your own. Maybe just save the money, as you pee them out anyway. So they can't be all that important then, right? Only an American Gothic would have a problem with that, wouldn't you agree?

But diet and supplementation are only two-thirds of the problem. Working out or lack thereof is still hanging out there for consideration. Some people don't do any kind of workout and most of those who do only put out with cell-phone-in-your-ear intensity, but you're shooting hoops with the kid and that's somethin', isn't it? That's more than the neighbor does, and it is like doing what the doc talked about a while back. So you're okay, right? In other words, who let the American Gothic in the back door?

Hopefully you aren't all this pathetic. But you may be, and that has to stop, tough as that may be. It's especially so when you're starting out at forty and have really never done any type of health-conscious living before. All Ms. D and I can say is that we respect your efforts (applaud them, in fact) as long as they are GOFHW efforts. And yes, I know this sounds austere, just like Gothic Americana.

In order for you to do hard workouts every day of the week, your diet will have to be top-notch. Then and only then might you actually be able to keep up the pace of everyday training. That is what you need to make this all work. You must really put out as you go through the motions and you must take the guilt seriously, even if you're just too sore or too tired to show up on day two. Missing that day only means you must make up what you miss over the next few days. That's what being serious all is about. It means being consistent, with no excuses, which requires that you stay away from those silly enough to believe in excuses (for your own good, of course) or, worse yet, who make the excuses *for* you.

Surely, this must all be sounding more and more Gothic by the sentence. How can anyone live like this in modernday America? Won't everyone stay away from you because we're making you into a Health Nut—somebody incapable of having fun? That almost sounds contradictory, doesn't it: a nut that isn't any fun to be around, when nuts are supposed to be all fun and games? It almost sounds as if no one will like me, if I do what this five-hundred-year-old guy and his wife say I should. Sounds like I'll look like I belong in the American Gothic picture as well!

We've tried getting you to stay away from these Normal Majority friends of yours at other points throughout the book. We've told you that it's safer standing in front of your own barn with a pitchfork than it is having coffee and donuts with them. But we know our warnings will never be enough. We know you've still got Normal Majority folks hanging around and you're still trying to fit right in with them. We even know how some of you brag to them about manipulating your doctor (how she just got out of med school with that wetness behind the ears). So that's where you're at, and that's that.

I know we are a bit radical. What we strongly believe in is not considered the norm. And yes, we would agree, we're not very friendly. There just really are some things that we cannot tolerate (which means we think they're not okay). Maybe you needn't be as harsh, but you will eventually need to reevaluate some the things that right now you feel are important.

I will never forget walking into a sports medicine clinic five years ago and remarking on an ad for an anti-cholesterol pill: "It's not you; it's your genes," it said. A young woman physician looked at me in an approving way for what she mistakenly thought was my sincere interest. As if someone had pulled her Chatty Cathy cord, she said, "Yes, so many are the product today of what they received from their relatives, and we as a culture, having been put so much emphasis on what we do as if its never enough, yada yada yada"—I stopped her and simply said, "My levels were up twenty points ten years ago, making me step up the aerobics and add more fiber. After one year, they were normal. You are more than welcome to check it right now if you'd like."

This did not go over well, as I'm sure you can imagine. Here she was, trying to help me with my problem, trying to make a monstrous excuse for me before even knowing whether I had a dietary or exercise reason to have high cholesterol, or if I even had it at all. She was willing to admit me to the Everyone Club, which is supposedly impacted across the board genetically by first- or second-tier relatives. Therefore, she was driven (talk about compulsion) to get me onto the latest wonder of modern science—yet another pill from one of the big drug manufacturers.

Granted, she was trying to be nice and not judgmental, but really her mindlessness was unforgivable. Without even checking me out, she had me diagnosed. Without even knowing if I was a slacker or a disciplined athlete, she knew that I needed help with my body chemistry. Someone might have been helped by this approach, but I didn't want it *ever* to be me. Not like that, I didn't!

Clearly, I didn't care to have her check my LDL levels to see if they might have gone up. What I was really telling her was to take down this silly poster, drop the enabler attitude, and start telling her patients to replace their full-time patienthood (or drug dependence) by becoming athletes.

This seemed wholly appropriate, as I was sitting in a sports medicine clinic that paid her salary. That's why I purposely said "athletes" instead of "healthy persons." Further, I made it clear by my demeanor that I was in no mood for a one-upping. "Aren't you being a bit harsh?" from a woman forty years my junior carrying twenty too many pounds was *not* going to happen.

Ms. D and I both think that the country ought to be outraged at any young medical professional not yet thirty who sounds like a TV ad. It's not so much that they are arrogant, but that they are such products of their environment, rather than critically free-thinking recent graduates of fine universities. Sure, she meant less harm than I did, but who do you think is right for the good of the country as whole?

Can it be that every medical problem has a genetic cause? I hope not, but who knows? More than likely, this clinic is not the only place we'll find the same set of attitudes. What's frightening is the ease with which the theory just rolls from their mouths, as if from an educated Chatty Cathy doll. That ought to be enough to keep everyone away from such professionals whenever possible.

You would have the courage to walk out on them before they got into doing your checkup and giving banal advice, wouldn't you? Or is that too American Gothic: pitch fork and sober expression?

You would walk out if you wanted to think of yourself, and maybe everyone else, as more than the product of your genes. You won't, if you think that being politically correct, being neither harsh nor rude, and blindly accepting the wonders of modern science are always good things. If that's where you are, you'll go right back for the same old snake oil to smooth away your troubles. You'll go back to the bright young MDs and politely listen as they let you off the hook for your laziness. Maybe her MD bosses will even turn up the soothing music in the background to make everything less painful. You may even believe that if you buy enough of their little pills for long enough, they will correct your problem, whatever it may be.

All well and good, we guess. But is that what you want? We doubt it, even if it is so demonstrative of the modern-day wonders of modern science. Americans really don't like being dependent on anything. We're the home of the brave and land of the free, folks, kind of like American Gothics standing in front of their bought-and-paid-for barn with a pitchfork, not afraid of GOFHW.

But it's true that we're also the land of the most technology. So which is better, when, why, and how? You are the one who has to make the final decision. Do you want to be the product of modern science's advances? If so, you will always be enthralled by the new wonders that emerge every month.

Some of these wonders really do eliminate the threat of conditions we used to fear. We admit it. So what's so bad about them? Well, maybe nothing, as long as they stay within the appropriate bounds, as long as they only treat what they're supposed to treat. But do you need to be treated? Are they really right for you? Or might GOFHW be just a little bit better? Be your own MD for a moment, and come up with an answer.

Conclusion

Do dare to be different.
Don't settle for the life of ease and quick fixes.

14

It's Never Too Late to Be Like Arnold

Any reasonable person should know that cutting back on sports activity when you're over the hill is wise, if not just plain mandatory. After all, you're not a kid anymore, now that you just turned fifty. Maybe you can do some laps of the track every other day or so at the club, but that should be it. Much more than that will get you sore muscles, or even pulled ones, which might make you walk a little strange for a day or two. That's why you shouldn't do anything more than every other day. More than that means you won't have a chance to recover. Of course, your waistline may get a little larger as a result of such a halfhearted effort, but why should you care? Better safe than injured, and "no love handles" is for high school kids. Do what's okay for circulation and heart, but skip the Olympic training. That's for the young guys (and girls, though not enough of them seem to think they are a Dara Torres). Besides, to be mature means accepting some of the hallmarks of growing older. That's what acting your age is all about, and everyone knows that that's what everybody ought to be doing.

Friends, if you believe all of this, we're never going to get along, and you're going to stay dumpy for the rest your days. You really need some new people to talk to (or you need to listen to us).

That's why it is so exciting when an article with a picture of a woman in her mid-seventies doing a weight workout appears on the bulletin board at the health club. Here is someone well over the age of thirty (by forty-five or more years, in fact) who hasn't bought into the have-a-nice-day society we've all come to accept as normal. Here she is, pumping iron at seventy-five, maybe eighty. And there's no grimace on her face.

Is this bad, weird, Health Nutty? Maybe to some, but Ms. D and I don't think so. That's what makes us different from the Normal Majority and their narc-like guardians, the FBI. That's why Ms. D and I start looking for snoops when we see articles about senior citizens pumping iron. We wonder when the bad guys will see this, tear it down, and go after the author. The seventy-five-year-old woman is safe, but the author of the article is not.

This may sound paranoid, but the thought of a trim, wrinkle-free super-retiree getting bikini-ready is just un-American. That's enough to attract FBI attention. Scoff if you must. But a woman in extraordinary shape and getting even more so when she should be frail and getting set for the nursing home does more than raise an eyebrow or two. The long-term care facility owners just might start getting uptight. Who knows, maybe even AARP would start looking even more tired out and ho-hum to more sixty-year-olds than it currently does, assuming that's even remotely possible. Where would they be if far fewer people consulted with them via their website, with its megahits? What if everyone who is really far over the forty hill started becoming like this lady and the incomparable nineties-plus LaLanne?

The Feds do monitor very left-wing political groups. They would prefer that this woman look saggy, wrinkly, and plump, and jovial at the thought of making a pumpkin pie for Thanksgiving. She is not supposed to look better than her daughter does. No elder-care products or programs would make sense if she did. Granted, her daughter may be a Miss America lookalike, so you can say that it runs in the family (great genes), but it's far more likely that her daughter looks the part of a burned-out mommy, not caring to work off her post-pregnancy pounds. Clearly, that's cruel to say, but how many are there like that nowadays? If this type of daughter had a mom who looked the iron woman part, their Thanksgiving dinners might really be very tense, wouldn't you think?

Jack LaLanne has irrefutably demonstrated that you can keep getting into better condition, which means getting biologically younger, as the years go on. This is heresy in relation to the orthodox aging paradigm that we have all grown up to accept. "You're not getting any younger" is what you are always told, and in ways that make it impossible not to believe. It's supposed to make you chuckle. You're getting closer to death with every birthday party, something you're supposed to enjoy. Sober maturity is the knowledge that you are getting older each day and that nothing, including you, lasts forever.

The spirit-killing implications of all of this are obvious. But the biggest killer is the dogmatic assertion that you can do nothing to stop it. That's the gospel (the dubious good news) that the Normal Majority never gets tired of preaching. But this is where LaLanne proves these degreeless experts wrong. He gets better by the year. The woman in the ad looks like she does likewise. What's even more encouraging is that her example shows that it can start happening for you, too, in just six months.

This is our message, plain and simple. You too can make significant changes in as little as six months. Her success is our justification for saying, "Start now and good things will happen, regardless of where you are or where you have been." Whether you are seventy or thirty-eight, you can start turning back the clock. But you have to be doing the right things, right now. It won't happen after just one swig of water from the fountain of youth, as the legend suggests, but it will after six months of hard, consistent low-fat, low-carb dieting, supplementation, and working out. That's little other than GOFHW, our fountain water for you in a bottle.

Certainly no one would doubt that the seventy-five-year-old in the picture did something very similar. Elderly people, if that word can even be used for her, are like that. They believe in discipline and hard work, wouldn't you agree? Is there a grandparent-type around who doesn't? Okay, maybe there are a few stragglers who don't, but that's not the norm, is it? Ms. D and I don't think so. Furthermore, neither you nor anyone else would ever accuse her of getting GH (growth hormone) injections, the mild-mannered relative of the steroid dianabol, for mature adults. (Though if she did, it should really be no worse than getting a Boniva shot like Sally Field talks about on TV. It shouldn't unless you think that shots for osteoporosis are okay, while shots for enhanced vitality are not.) Discipline and consistency are part of maturity in over-sixty adults. So this woman is believable. She regularly lifted weights, and they made her look great.

By contrast, the Bowflex machine (frequently on TV ads) didn't make the twenty-seven-year-old model look the way she does, or at least Ms. D and I strongly doubt it. If you have seen these ads on TV, you know that the Bowflex works wonders. Of course, as GOFHW people, we don't think it does unless you keep at it for a couple of years in conjunction with some other things. Rather, we think her natural youthfulness did what the Bowflex people want you to think their equipment did.

Okay, maybe she had done some training for some time, but how much are we talking about, really? Not even a thousandth of what LaLanne or Torres did. You would agree with that even without writing each of them, wouldn't you? Besides, we're talking about attitudes here, not clinical studies. It's what you do with what you're confronted with that matters most.

I throw this in because the research institute that did the study on weight training and aging compared genetic samplings from other seventy-five-year-olds and some much younger people. The seventy-five-year-olds who had done weight training were biologically younger than the younger folks who had done nothing. Perhaps the seventy-five-year-old did not have the cellular structure of a twenty-seven-year-old, but what if it were that of a forty-six-year-old? That would still be dramatic enough, wouldn't it?

Ms. D and I do not doubt these findings. Someone from the University of Common Sense might think that everybody should be cynical about them ("They must be sellin' somethin'"), but we aren't. This is largely because we are different from people our chronological age, and we know why.

We trained ardently by the decade, meaning that we never hung it up when everybody thought we should. But we are not the only ones who are like this. Tests that measure biological age have been around for at least a decade. If you haven't seen any of these, you might tomorrow when you check your e-mails, finding a new longevity product that claims to turn back the clock. Antioxidants are pretty much all like this. The accompanying studies suggest that there are real cellular changes that can be experienced and be measured.

Those studies will enrage the Normal Majority, who are convinced that nothing does anything to ever change their bodies for the better after age thirty (explaining the jokes about becoming thirty-something). The number of these folks is overwhelming. This group is far too dignified to ever be accused of being Health Nuts. At least, that's what they seem to be all about all of the time. They would never let their hair down to try something like Mangosteen, a great-tasting antioxidant. That's all a lot of hokum; it won't *ever* work, as they know. Even when it makes them feel better almost immediately, it's just because of the suggestion that it would give them a lift (the placebo effect).

You may be one of these normal folks, though your purchase of this book suggests that you are not. Some people just refuse to give up hope, even though the Normal Majority thinks this is what makes you a Health Nut. Sound like you? According to them, some poor adolescent types won't ever stop looking for Ponce DeLeon's fountain. How young can ya get? That's why they are compelled to say that they've tried all that and it just doesn't work. It's better to be mature than joyful. That's not you, is it?

What needs to be addressed is not so much studies like those that accompany anti-aging products or the article about the seventy-five-year-young weightlifter, but what people do with them before they investigate or even begin to think about them. Today, we expect that most folks will put these studies in the circular file cabinet of frivolous stuff the Health Nuts get off on, meaning not part of mainstream medical science. In other words, they go into a place with other purely academic junk that truly does not speak to real people. This is like the supposed frivolity of the supercollider, which will enable scientists to understand the first milliseconds of the universe's inception. How will that knowledge help with the national debt? You get the picture, right? That translates to saying that real science should not waste its time on such frivolity as getting Grandma bikini-perfect by July. Any research money for this purpose ought to go elsewhere, where it's needed.

Politicians, the elected spokespeople of the Normal Majority, think money should go for studies having to do with a cure for diabetes, heart disease, and so on. Considering the fact that these folks have constituents who frequently get diagnosed with high blood sugar and the like, it most certainly will. Forget the wishful thought that you wouldn't have to cure all of these people if you turned them into middle-aged athletes earlier on. Oh no. That's way too Health Nutty, isn't it? After all, we are supposed to know by now that an ant just can't move a rubber tree plant, and all that.

The sad thing is that the article about the woman in her seventies was on the bulletin board at the club for about two days. Someone took it down, and there is no way to know why. Was it taking up too much space? Perhaps. Who knows, except for the person who took it down,; and considering how unreflective so many folks are, they themselves might not even know. But we can guess it's because it was deemed not interesting to enough people. There is an overabundance thirty- to fifty-year-olds who work out there. None of these could care about a real person who's old enough to be their mother pumping iron, could they? Probably not.

They are probably all much more interested in the twenty-seven-year-old Bowflex model lookalike and the absurd wistful belief that they could never be her equal. Oh, to be young again … sigh. We, of course, think they could, if only they would start today, but that makes us out to be some real radicals, I'm sure.

But can the Normal Majority understand any of this in that way? In other words, could they say, "There but for grace of GOFHW go I?" I don't think so, do you? Just as you can't fight city hall, you can't think for yourself when the media along with that AMA and all of common sense are against you.

Making it to seventy-five is good; making it to eighty is even better. No one ever says in what form, but it is presumed that okay-form means good enough to lift the fork at Thanksgiving dinner and maybe tell an after-dinner story about the good old days—but that's it! No one, absolutely no one expects, or would even tolerate, a story from a seventy-five-year-old about lifting more this month than her grandson did as an undergrad (no matter how tactfully said). The same goes for running one mile in pretty close to five and a half minutes. Such people would be in the freak category, which is very similar to being in the Health Nut category. And that, my friends, is not where anyone wants to be.

There is nothing to support what I am going to assert, but my feeling is that a grandparent who is in super shape would have kids and grandkids who would spend a whole year finding a way to not invite this iron person, a seventy-five-year-old hard body, to next year's Thanksgiving dinner. And that's in spite of their anticipated positions in the will! So you know this must be serious.

How they would pull off not inviting them is a bit of a mystery at present, but my guess is that it would involve inanities such as just not having the time or money this year to do what we'd like for turkey day. That might solve the problem for this coming year, and maybe that will be enough, assuming Grandma just may have a heart attack after doing s marathon in Duluth.

You think that I am overdoing it? You think that nobody would snub Mom or Grandma for something like this? Dream on. Parents get put into the strange category and are treated as inhuman if they do not fit the mold—the mold made for them by their kids and a host of meddling others. It's not the one they choose. They pick up designations like "old girl," "old boy," or "character." These are all variations of the senile-variety Health Nut. They're fringy, marginal—off to the side instead of in the center where we all want to be.

What should happen is that these sixty-plus beach-perfect parents ought to simply get disgusted with their kids and say something like, "You never did do what was reasonable when you were young, so why should anyone hope for more now?"

Then they should make plans with their own like-minded friends for next year's Thanksgiving. That way they can avoid the heavy meal and be too busy to go with their supportive loved ones. But will any of this happen?

Probably not, and that is really too bad. One year of not having them there might cause enough guilt to get the thirty-somethings into some better living habits as well as becoming duly respectful of their betters.

The point is that things are not the way that they ought to be. Any sensational seventy-five-year-old flaunting her hundred-and-fifty-pound bench press at a Thanksgiving dinner will be considered a problem instead of an inspiration. The kids will get uptight, as will the rest of the in-laws. That ought not to be, but it will, unless something starts happening now.

That's why it's time for you and me to stick together to stop this snobbery throughout the US of A, the land of the free and brave—or is the land of complacency and paunchiness? We need to start in February saying a grace which gives thanks for Grandma having done so much for herself as an iron woman, and thus for all of us. Then Thanksgiving might be associated with some welcome changes.

Conclusion

Do pump iron even if you're seventy.
Don't slow down just to keep your kids happy.

15

Take Hold and Take Charge

The "Let go and let God" attitude (the opposite of the "Take Hold and Take Charge" one) of the person growing old gracefully is something that God would never approve of. The people who age gracefully (any age will do here as long as you're doing the mature thing of letting go) think that nature does everything significant. That is the biggest part of the problem.

This is the reason that Ms. D and I get treated like Health Nuts when we try to help people with their waistlines. In a tough-love fashion, we tell them they are sagging and that it's their fault that they are. What we're really saying is that they have to *do* something about it. But our accusations understandably don't win us many friends, even among those who say that they want things to be different. Presumably, we are supposed to say that sagging just kind of happens as you age, and that's okay. Now doesn't that sound like something you'd expect to read on the AARP website?

That is all well and good, and maybe that's what should be said to those in nursing homes nearing the end of their lives. But is that you? Perhaps the really old folks are even afflicted by a life-sapping illness such as cancer. Folks like this do not need to hear about how much more they should or could be doing to maximize their physical potential. Instead, they need to be left off the hook so they can comfortably enjoy the few days they may have left. In other words, it would be a thoughtlessly cruel thing to suggest that their conditions could be improved by their running ten miles every day, or completely pointless to say that possibly they wouldn't be sick in the first place if only they had started training earlier on. No one who is badly off should have to hear anything like that. But again, is that you? Are you so close to the end of your days that you ought not to hear our "Get with it, before *it* gets you?"

All adults should know that there are things in life far more important than looking good in a Speedo or bikini. Assuming that you are over forty, we really can't imagine you disagreeing with that. Having been granted the minimum level of good health (meaning that all of your vital signs are the way they should be in addition to good cholesterol levels with no peripheral arterial symptoms) after forty should be enough. Presumably, no one in their right mind should be demanding more. Think of those poor folks in Africa. We have it great here in the US, and that should be enough for anyone. Thus saith the Normal Majority.

So no one should demand more—perhaps. No one should unless it's you for yourself, of course. Then the question can become "Do you want something more, something that's maybe a little gutsy?" You know what we mean. We're thinking of a sophisticated version of grabbing all the gusto you can (from a beer commercial from a few years back) without having the energy immediately drain away after some sudden bursts of vitality.

What we're talking about is that quiet, boundless reserve type of energy in a fat-free form, which enables you to be ready to enjoy movement whenever and wherever you might like. Then all you need to do is to throw in a little of that movie-star appeal and you've got it. That's what we're all after, isn't it? It's like being on cruise control all day at 70 mph when your car is capable of 120 mph without overheating. It's just like being the way you were when you were back in high school. Or have you never experienced this even when younger, so you don't even know how great *great* is?

Clearly, this is a rather worldly and with-it form of enjoying your life. It's not at all like the very quiet saint-like wasting away that seniors so often get into in a very contemplative and dignified fashion. Rather, it's very much like being the driver of your car on cruise control, almost completely free to enjoy the ride. It's all about you directing where you are going and just letting the computer adjust the fuel and air intake. That keeps the motor at a constant speed, enabling you to cruise through the weekends and vacations if you're younger, or cruise through your retirement if you're older.

Some folks think this is letting go and letting God. But that is entirely different. Letting go in the much-used sense means that you are not at the wheel. Instead, either God or nature is. That's more like you being the passenger, sitting back while waiting for something to happen, like maybe an accident or running out of gas. That's precisely what can occur when you are no longer in control, when someone else is doing the driving, and that can be true at forty or at eighty.

Being on cruise control is what we should all be after. You do this on the highway on a long, easy trip, looking at beautiful scenes out the window, so you know what we mean. Not only is this different from leaving the driving to someone else, but it is the complete opposite of the stressful stop-and-go driving in the city, made even worse when you're close to empty (the presumed end of your days at eighty in the Normal Majority's mind). This is when you can get rear-ended, hit a curb, or run out of fuel at almost any time.

But most folks are not this harried unless they are living with a ticking clock thinking their time is running out. That is a problem for modern science in the case of dread diseases, or a psychologist in the case of unconsciously contrived limits.

Our goal is to turn passengers into drivers on cruise control. That's what diet, supplementation, and working out ought to be all about, whatever your chronological age. We think that there is more that can be done with a life than merely taking a long, much deserved rest—after a whole week of work for those in their mid-forties, or a whole life of work for those in their seventies. (If you are exhausted just reading this, our advice is that what we're promoting is most probably not for you. In that case, you might want to check with a doctor.)

We are all about creating vitality. Therefore, when the Normal Majority thinks you ought to be taking time off with a large supply of martinis in Cancun, or becoming serene enjoying your place in the Ft. Lauderdale sun, we think you ought to be out running five miles. Skip the baking away while doing nothing, even if the travel posters make that look so great. Sell your thermosful of booze to the people on the blanket next to you and buy some green tea and mega-multivitamins with the proceeds.

To some, this may sound just too much like there's never any rest for the wicked. That's pretty much why the Normal Majority thinks we're almost sacrilegious. They may have a point, but try not knocking our thing until you've tried it.

All we can say is that peace on earth, good will to all humankind is truly more important than auditioning for *Baywatch*. It's just that we don't see how giving up the dream of looking good on the beach at fifty-five, or even walking about in a saintly fashion if you are seventy-five, makes you better able to love your neighbor—or God, for that matter. In fact, we think that making such a renunciation at thirty-five or forty, like most folks do (in the name of being adults) makes you a rather angry person later, prone to all sorts of unhappy thoughts, feelings, and activities.

But, that's for psychologists to elaborate upon, and maybe for those closest to you—the ones who have to endure your endless discontentment. All we know is that everything goes better when you're supplementing, exercising, and eating right and that those effects start within the first sixty days regardless of where you've been before. It's that dynamic, poised humanity look instead of a worn-out one that we're talking about.

We think that anyone can do the graceful aging routine, acting more like a kindly grandparent every day, as long as they work at it. It's not hard. It's all part of acting your age, something that the Normal Majority thinks you always ought to be doing, assuming you're up there in *that* age bracket (whatever it is). All you have to do is cooperate with all of the little signs that seem to prove that you aren't as young as you used to be. The easiest to identify are those little tired periods that most folks misinterpret as the advent of an impending total slowdown. You are supposed to embrace them as if they are the welcomed handwriting on the wall. The belief is that cooperating with them will enable you to stick around as long as possible.

Our trouble with these little energy slowdowns is that they are no different from the same minor lags at other points in your life, like maybe when you were sixteen. Take a few moments to think back. We've all had them. The easiest to remember are the ones you used to take advantage of, such as playing hooky from school or needing a mental holiday to recover from too much stress. It's just that now you're supposed to take them all so seriously because you really are over forty—the *big 4 oh*. In other words, you're not as young as you used to be, like when you were thirty-nine!

Friends, you can really throw your self into this supposedly Sensible Slowdown Syndrome, the SSS, if you'd like, but you won't impress us in the process. You'll probably turn on your minister, your friends, relatives, and neighbors, but none of these, I assure you, will include Ms. D and me. Unless you're suffering from some disease for which you are probably on a powerful antibiotic, this is an absurdity.

We believe that there is a near bottomless well of potential inside everyone. This is like the motor that can go 120 mph if it has to, but cruises easily all day at 70 mph. That means there's still way too much inside that's simply not getting worked with. And why is that? It is because you're walking around acting your age to keep all of your Normal Majority critics happy. And of course, you're just not working out, dieting, and supplementing the way you should. As a result, you are turning into a kindly grandparent.

Perhaps you think that it is wonderful being a nice warm grandparent who is sought after by his or her grandchildren. But what age are we talking about: eighty-five, ninety, or forty-five going on ninety-two? The example of LaLanne immediately comes to mind. He's up there at ninety-five this year, but doesn't look the part. He does a two-hour workout every day and promotes his juicer. He is not like anyone else who's up there with him "down under," like at seventy-five!

So should we feel sorry for him? Don't laugh. Maybe we should. Maybe he's like all the overachievers. If so, he's at a complete disadvantage when it comes to normal relationships. Maybe that's painful. Maybe his family doesn't like him. Maybe; but his wife is pretty cute and the twenty-eight-year-old who helped him market his juicer recently did not have close to his energy level.

We think there are far too many people acting the part of grandparents when in fact they're really far more dynamic. The trouble is that the more they try to fit this mold, the more they slow down and actually become it. The hard part for us is seeing this and not being able to do anything about it, because these people see themselves as being so well adjusted and blessed by such wonderful kids and grandkids. How can we scoff at that without appearing to be monsters?

All too often, we see the start of acting grown up, mature, dignified (really being your age) as incongruent and thus no more than an act. It starts out as a wet blanket on a flame, and in a short while the blanket completely takes over the entire person. Then the acting is over and the diminished vitality is completely where it's at. If only people would do the grandma and grandpa thing out in public, kind of like an act or charade, and then quickly change into their track clothes for a ten-mile run, the world would be a better place. But that never happens.

Of course, psychologically, it can't. People just are not this way when it comes to major identity issues like these. People act real because they are for real and want to be seen that way by everyone. Therefore, they proudly take the grandparent identity to heart, slowing themselves down completely, proving to themselves and others that they are very okay, if not just a little bit short of glorious.

Our biggest problem with the graceful agers is that the effects of this are relatively sudden and irreversible. Talk about an extreme makeover! That's what happens when you let yourself go. You and everyone around you can see it almost overnight, just like they can the effects of diet, exercise, and supplementation. It is allowed to happen, probably because you now think it's time. Then everything inside you changes. Given another sixty days, you can see the differences in the mirror. So can everyone else as well.

We are taught to believe that taking it easy is the best thing for everyone—everyone over the age of thirty, that is. Prior to this point, you are supposed to be full of beans—the fruit that does little more than make you toot. Being mature means putting all of this farting about aside with a "been there, done that." Sorry if that's offensive, but that type of verbiage is why the mature, dignified adult masses sit on their increasingly unsightly asses instead of competing in marathons. It's kid stuff.

Our question is "Are you really all that worn out and in need of a break from having to put out at the gym, or are you acting that way to appease your friends, relatives, and neighbors—the Normal Majority?" Maybe the next question should be "Can you be honest with yourself and come up with an authentic answer when it comes to where you really are?" You may be too afraid of the consequences of being in shape to be able to pull it off. Maybe it's too much of a risk. But it's a risk of what? Being called a Health Nut instead of a worn-out adult (a graceful ager)? Sticks and stones … you know the rest.

The Normal Majority believes that the ills of celebrating birthdays are inevitable. You can't avoid them. They're just like death and taxes, heh, heh, heh (in witch-cackle fashion). That's maturity, so they believe. That is the way it is. That's ultimate reality; forget what all of the Health Nuts from Leon think. You can't live forever, you're going to die, and that's that!

We think that attitudes like these do far more to slow a person down than do any of the natural processes inside them. We know of people who are in their sixties and in better shape than they were in high school. The big difference between them and the Normal Majority is that they made decisions to not cooperate with any of the supposedly sure signs that they had just gotten old. Those little lags that we all experience never are anything more to them than just that. They are the same today at sixty as when you got a tummy ache in grade school. They aren't indicative of the handwriting being on the wall.

We think that if after forty-five you are doing as expected by expanding at the middle, it must be that you are taking the car when you could be walking, doing the Internet when you could be jogging, talking to your wife on the cell phone in the car when you could both be briskly walking after a dinner of salad with chicken and tofu. You also must be getting happier than ever by way of celebrating on TGIF, drinking an increasing number of Buds while watching the game(s), and regularly downing a half a box of chocolates while reading yet another cheap novel. These are the activities you're expected to be into in addition to frequenting McDonald's every weekend as a reward for all of the Monday through Friday sacrifices.

All of that is well and good. Praise to the Normal Majority! But these are the activities that make your inner life force a four-cylinder engine with one of the valves plugged instead of a glorious V-8.

As there are so many encouragements from the media, you will have an easy time doing these things. In fact, it will be a compulsion, although the Normal Majority would never approve of calling it that. (Compulsiveness is for Health Nuts, you see.) But the fact is that you will be driven to do the okay thing. It will feel normal; it is expected; it's what everybody does and everybody, namely your kids, knows what to expect. They'll get a washed-out older person to be nice to them and their kids. They'll get their moms and dads at predictable holiday get-togethers with lots of good stroking. What they won't get is the discomfort at having to sit next to someone twice their age who is prepping for the senior iron person's competition!

Ms. D and I are convinced that most folks do not really know what they are capable of. They know what will happen if they dare to step out of the roles they're expected to play and the people they're expected to be. They don't know what could be better than fitting into the categories their kids and the media put them into. Maybe that means there is nothing else, or this is as good as it gets? The Normal Majority believes that this is the way it is. Nevertheless, you may have a desire for something different, which is why you bought this book.

There are no easy, attractive answers to training like champions. There are only dry, repetitive ones, ones that no one likes. There is no wonder pill. Everything that sounds easy, as if it could fit into the fast-food immediate gratification category, is doomed. It's hype—something to get you to buy something.

The good news is that all you really need is good old-fashioned hard work and discipline: GOFHW, nothing more. It will work eventually regardless of where you start, whether at forty-five or seventy. It will turn your inner energy reserve into a V-8 engine. and it will do this even if right now it's a four hittin' on three and you're driving a clunker. But it won't do so overnight. All that can be said is that working at it while everybody else is trying to fit into their kids' expectations will ultimately do the trick.

The bad news is that GOFHW work is hard. It's not a lot of fun. At least it isn't until you really get into it. Thus, anyone who wants to hold you back for whatever reason can do a pretty good job of scaring you out of doing it.

That's the truth, and it just might be the best reason to find and enjoy some new friends who don't keep telling you to take it easy. Maybe it's time to find them now and turn over a new leaf. What could be so bad about that? After all, they, too, might have nowhere to go for Thanksgiving dinner.

Conclusion

Do get yourself on cruise control.
Don't be afraid of 70 mph at seventy years young.

16

How Much Is Just Right?

How much is too much? How much is not enough? These are two ways of getting at the same thing, but neither is very helpful, even if we know we're talking about revolutions per minute and poundage, when it comes to you specifically. What kind of an Iron Person do you want to become? That really is your call, you know—or maybe you don't. Anyway, there are different kinds, and you have a choice. But the point is that we have to know what we're really talking about to make any sense out of a question like this.

So what is right? Is an hour of exercise daily just right, too much, or not enough? Then do you do it at a particular level of resistance or at a certain number of rpms? Is it the same for a person starting out as it is for someone who's been at it for a whole three weeks? What about someone who is 180 pounds in relation to one who is 130? What about body type and muscularity? What about being a man or a being a woman?

A right amount, it seems, should somehow be impacted by all of these considerations, if not some others as well. But they should all be subordinate to the big two questions:

- ❖ What are you really up to? or
- ❖ What are you trying to make happen for yourself?

How many people ask questions of this type when it comes to working out, supplementation, and dieting?

How many people really want what they say they want? Let's say that the final answer to that question may take some time and a lot of rethinking, so let us make an offer in the here and now. Maybe we can come up with kind of a *basic* newbie.

Ms. D and I are most interested in hearing that you want to become fat free, free-breathing, energetic, optimistic, and attractive enough to be envied at the beach by people from places like the PTA and church. That is hardly the same as frequenting a dimly lit bar, where most of our over-forty married readers would never go anyway. Many folks, realizing that we are interested in getting you to look great for the summer (in other words, a fabulous forty or fifty or a sensational sixty or seventy), might be inclined to completely write us off if we didn't say this. But becoming beach ready for every summer from now on until you really are too old to even see a beach in your imagination is probably the only thing that will make you do what you must to maximize your healthiness. In short, doin' it for Doctor, even if it's to stave off diabetes, just won't cut it for the long haul; doing it for your own self-esteem and your spouse's happiness *will.*

Therefore, you would do well to stifle your sanctimonious pseudo-stoicism (if you feel yourself getting a tad prissy right now) and just realize that you will not lapse into self-destroying (sinful) vanity by getting to like what you see in the mirror. Experience should have shown you that long ago, but Mom and/or Dad may have made you phobic when it comes to self-love. If that sounds like where you've been, try to get beyond it right now. Surely you would agree that nothing very bad will happen if you occasionally give yourself kudos for your appearance and let yourself have some respectable peer admirers. All we can say is that if this makes you feel a little vain, try it anyway and see if being really healthy doesn't make it all go away in three to four months or so.

If you are really okay with the ideas we're trying to put into your head, you have some new habits to pick up. A personal transformation from couch potato to *Baywatch* auditioner will require some ongoing care. You will have to change your living habits—that is, your life. So get with it. Some people think this will entail a lot. But it doesn't really have to unless you're going to make a big deal (drama) out of the drudgery of going to the club, giving up the thick, juicy steaks, downing all of those pills. Friends, all you have to do is do supplement, eat properly, and exercise. Nothing much else is required unless you want to throw in these: drink enough filtered water (as chlorine is problematic, as is the other stuff that's in tap water), get enough sleep, and deal with stress. All are good ideas and hardly rocket science, right? We're sure you'd agree.

But let's get back to "How much is enough?" as a general question. Our rational answer is that we don't know for sure, but that's only because we're not you. Yet we know more than your standard advice-giver: the person who thinks he or she knows something from reading a training manual or textbook so special that it's never available at Barnes & Noble or Borders. You know more, too, even if you don't really know it yet.

What we're saying is that you should systematically use your own head. That means keeping track of what you do in a log or diary (and looking back at your entries every Saturday) while using the seek-and-ye-shall-find method. Thus you should start with, let's say, one hour of cycling on level three of your club's many (empty) exercycles. Then you should ask yourself if you can do this again tomorrow with the idea of never missing for a year. If the answer is "No way," then you cut back to level two. If it's "I don't feel like I did anything on three at all," then maybe you should increase it to level four. That's the seek-and-ye shall-find method, which you use until you reach and maintain an optimal level of performance.

The beauty of this method lies in its inexpensiveness and self-sufficiency. You needn't consult first with your MD. Nevertheless, if the mere thought of doing this level of exercise is exhausting, then you probably are not okay physically and may really need that trip to your doctor to ask if exercise is right for you. (Is the FBI reading? See, I sent them to the doctor, so I'm not all bad—I mean radical.) But is this really where you're at? If not, skip the consultation. That will save you time and money and us a ton of aggravation.

Moreover, you can skip the personal trainer. They cost megadollars and seldom even think to work with you to come up with a good "how much?" answer for you because it says what's right in the book they use, and that's that. It's cheaper and better to get a book (like this one that you're reading maybe) that looks good to you and actually study it with you—as a person, not just a body—in mind.

In short, thinking about what you're doing while monitoring what you're doing, and then checking back over your notes once a week, will take you the farthest toward where you need to go. Yet some will still be uneasy about something so ... so, what. Truly grown up perhaps. Objective. Methodical. Scientific. Or did you mean to say scary?

If you are afraid to venture forth, play it safe and sure by being (Mickey Mouse) mature. Don't do anything until after your next doctor visit two months down the road, perhaps. The Normal Majority will respect you for that. All of your friends will, except us. We think that this kind of self-imposed restriction is just an excuse for not starting today, unless you're really too broken down, or God knows what.

There were no doctor visits for anything back where we came from in Leon. We had to take our own risks, just as we did when setting sail for Florida to not only get away from all of our dumpy friends, relatives, and neighbors but also to find the Fountain (so we told everyone). We did it. Why can't you? Yet there may be some really good reason.

The prevalent opinion in the last fifty years has been that rest and relaxation are the healthiest thing for the standard American citizen. Maybe this is so. Maybe everybody has worked too hard for too long and needs one big twenty-year vacation from vigorous living (retire at sixty-five, die at eighty-five, or work hard for five days so that you can pig out and relax for the next two). But we really think that taking this resting-up-so-that-you-can-die-better to heart has made Main Street America look awful.

Presumably, only a Health Nut would care about something so cosmetic how Main Street America looks. Isn't overall healthiness far more important? According to the Normal Majority, dumpiness is a small price to pay for healthiness, if it's even as bad as we're making it out to be in the first place. At least we're all safe, so they say. Presumably, that's only because we have the big folks watching over us to slow us all down to a nearly complete halt. How restfully wonderful, wouldn't you agree?

In other words, we supposedly need to be saved from bopping 'til we drop. Were it not for the wise counsel of those doctor folks with the two Mercedes who have too many patients to be free to work out, apparently we'd be hurting ourselves in droves. That's why with no—absolutely no— good statistical support (like they'd demand from us for our assertions), the Normal Majority ardently believes that none of us have the good sense to pace ourselves.

The perception is that any amount of sustained exertion is too much. Ask anyone over forty-five who has ever talked with his friends, relatives, and neighbors about working out. This includes, but is not limited to, a beginner's routine that you could (and should) start working on today. In other words, it includes really seeing if level three on the exercycle leaves you feeing like you've had a real workout and can do it all again tomorrow, Tuesday, not Wednesday (assuming today is Monday). Just that experimenting might be too much of a strain, and then where would you be? Oh my!

There have been signs on machines at health clubs in the past telling you to cut back if you start breathing heavily or sweating profusely. Thankfully, these skull-and-crossbones warning signs have been becoming less prevalent lately. In their places are pictures of how to do the exercise the machine was made for and the muscles which will be affected. This is helpful for those who lack the imagination needed to figure this out on their own. So things are improving, possibly? Our fingers are crossed. There may be a new tendency to view machines as your friends instead of your enemies, but we don't want to get too optimistic.

Generally, health clubs have people on staff to assist the newbies. Actually, they think they are there even to assist Ms. D and me, though they can't do half of what we can do. We do our best to be polite, but quite frankly, we are probably just plain rude. Maybe we should chill a bit, but we previously confessed to being American Gothics. After all, the folks we're talking about are compulsive helpers, always helping whether it's a good idea or not. Anyway, assuming you think their textbook authors all know more about you than you do, you can be assured that there will be an answer or two forthcoming—should you make the mistake of letting on that you might not know something.

But these people and books aren't your only resources. You can always ask people near you who look like they know what they're doing. That really can help if you haven't got the foggiest idea what to do, though we've never seen club members who would invest the time in extensively helping anybody with anything. Nevertheless, they may blurt out something quite helpful, as you've made them feel like Rocky for having asked.

All we can say is the same thing we always say: it's better to use your head than ask a bunch of questions of anyone. But you should first think of the machines as friends. That's far superior to showing up for a session with a trainer and worrying about what can happen to you if you overdo it.

You are supposed to think you haven't an ounce of good sense when it comes to working out. That is, you are expected to believe that you can't know yourself well enough to figure how many reps you need on each of the nautilus machines, and that you'll be completely befuddled when it comes to how much resistance on the bike, for example. "You can't know what you're doing," saith the Normal Majority. So now you know how to act, right?

Ms. D and I think this is hokum. Yet you need to have some thinking going on to make good on what we're saying. The seek-and-ye-shall-find method is best, but it should be influenced by some other things kept in the back of your mind. In other words, there are some benchmarks that you might want to consider. None are written in stone, yet they may help in your thought process. So get out a pen and some paper. Here goes:

- ❖ 20 reps to slim down
- ❖ 10 reps for overall conditioning
- ❖ 8 reps for shaping
- ❖ 6 reps for bulking up (only for halfbacks and muscle men)
- ❖ 3 reps for brute strength (something no one should be into, for some unknown reason)

Doing any or all of these every other day, never every day, is considered not only safest but completely best, as the muscles need a full forty-eight hours to recover. Doing more than this presumably results in atrophy, pain, pulled muscles, exhaustion, and susceptibility to illness, to say nothing about turning you into a gym rat (or muscle-bound).

Where did all of this come from? Ancient Greece? Unlikely. How about 1960s Kansas? We aren't sure, but we'd opt for the latter. If you believe that the sculptures are any indication of the way real Greeks looked back then, you might wonder what kinds of workout routines and diets they were into. Archaeological finds suggest that they were on very high-protein diets, but we have not as yet unearthed any further training specifications. Most likely, there were no exercise machines, yet given their advanced culture and architecture, who knows?

The point is that there was a long dark age between then and now. Possibly the "health renaissance" started with the TV appearances and exercise inventions of Jack LaLanne in the early 1960s and Jane Fonda in the early 1970s. In other words, our wisdom has come from the last forty years (though, sadly, it does not necessarily include much of Jack's or Jane's wisdom) and is really more in the form of *do not* than *do*. So where does that leave us? In 1960s Kansas or in 1960s Minnesota (where Ms. D and I have lived the most years since leaving Leon)?

Who knows, and who has time to do a whole lot of caring? None of us are into writing or reading about the history of physical conditioning, so let's just get with what's around in the here and now. Ms. D and I think you should start browsing health magazines at the supplement store. After three or four, you will pretty much get the drift of what everybody who knows anything seems to be doing in modern-day America. Granted, you won't be in the "three sets of four bent-over rows with 450 pounds" category like Arnold, but you certainly will fit into some other sensibly healthy category. Furthermore, you needn't be a bodybuilder to benefit. There are running magazines, *Men's Health* and *Women's Health* alongside the wannabe-just-like-Arnold ones. Take a look at some of those and you can go from there.

In other words, you should peruse magazines like these to get a feel for what you could and should be doing. They typically have articles about trim people in their forties: in other words, not just eighteen-inch bicep twenty-year-olds alongside silicone-boobed starlets! Regularly reading articles about these everyday healthy people and what they're doing is what the whole country should do. In our judgment, that's head and shoulders above thinking that maybe you should but not really knowing, and then after a few months asking your doctor if exercise is right for you.

In addition to twenty to thirty minutes a day of weight training, Ms. D and I think that you should do at least a half hour to forty-five minutes of aerobic something (cycling, hiking, jogging, or swimming) and do it every day with no excuses. You don't find any excuses for not brushing your teeth, so—fill in the blank. *Where is the issue?* Training is just like taking care of your teeth. If you want to have healthy teeth, you brush and floss them. If you want a dazzling smile, you go out of your way to get the best toothpaste and a battery-operated brush. And if you want to look good on the beach, you aerobically exercise, throw in some weight training, find a favorite brand of supplements (without complaining about having to swallow so many pills), and really get into healthy eating. This means continually finding favorite healthy meals so you are not forever moping about not getting to have any real food: steaks, pies, beers, and the like. That's what you do. Simple. No big deal. It's nothing more. Just do it as a matter of fact and leave all of the drama to your friends, relatives, and neighbors, who are card-carrying members of the Normal Majority.

So, friends, it's simple. Physical training is just like two minutes of brushing your teeth twice per day with a battery-operated toothbrush: the same song, second verse. It's just that when it comes to workouts, you have to invest more time. You do sixty minutes working out, meaning forty-five minutes of running and fifteen minutes on the weights machines. Then you shower off and dress. This you do every day, even on Christmas Day and your birthday. No issues. No excuses. No drama. Put that together with diet and supplements and you're good to go. Simple. That will keep you as good as new forever.

Conclusion

Do think for yourself when it comes to planning your diet, supplementation, and exercise routine.
Don't ever skip a day for any reason whatsoever.

17

From "I Didn't Know" to "A-Ha!"

It is incredible to think that someone can really *not* know that working out, supplementing, and eating a low-fat, low-carb diet will make significant physical changes. But there are a lot of folks who fall into this category. Their commonplace, surprised, and sonorous "I didn't know" (which was a line from two big drug company commercials not very long ago—one for the little purple pill, the other for an HPV med) is almost comical!

In its most usual form, "I didn't know" comes up as soon as a very healthy person indirectly confronts someone such as a prediabetic Normal Majority person with the simple truth that he could have done something to prevent his problem. This will happen in the form of a question like "Why didn't you just start exercising, supplementing, and eating correctly a long time ago?" They will then say, "*I didn't know* that any of those would be of any help."

Is this believable? Can it really be that so many have no idea of how to get truly healthy? Friends, hang on to your hats! Ms. D and I think so. That is, we believe that an incredible number of Americans are really, truly, wholeheartedly in the dark. They don't realize that doing the right things can be good for them. As strange as this may sound, as counter to all of the articles on the Internet, as completely opposite to the examples of people like Dara Torres and Jack LaLanne, it seems that we are living in a nation of people who really just *don't know*.

Nevertheless, in this very same country, some folks actually do wake up one morning saying, "I don't have to be like this." That's the same as saying, "Now, for once, I really *do* know" (that what they have played down is really worthwhile). In a land of unspeakable ignorance when it comes to real healthiness, the sudden change of heart is astonishing. Why? Because it comes from nowhere, straight out of the blue. "I didn't know" turns into "Now I can see."

How do people suddenly get so smart? This is curious, to put it mildly. We are all most comfortable with gradual progressions, and are in the habit of considering radical turnabouts highly suspect. We look for the other shoe to fall or for the new convert (a product of spontaneous remission, which the MDs all trust for some unknown reason) to become susceptible to a fatal relapse in the most extreme form of becoming broadsided. But what we *expect* and what *is* are two different things. Radical changes really do simply occur. Just as the bad things the down-and-outs say just happen, do happen, so do the good things. Sometimes, when these good things occur, they're followed by a sudden disdain for the harmless pursuits of real living. These include, but are not limited to, irritations about:

❖ Going out for donuts (the deep-fried and thus real variety, of course)
❖ Celebrating each TGIF with a cheeseburger blowout (after a whole week of putting up with the wholly unreasonable boss)
❖ Thinking Arby's (when you should be thinking Dannon yogurt)
❖ Letting stay in Vegas whatever happens in Vegas (that you shouldn't have gotten into in the first place)
❖ Thinking all of the Olympic athletes are on steroids (despite tests to the contrary)
❖ And finally, laughing at the Ms. America pageants (when there isn't one iota's worth of understanding of how hard she trains on a daily basis)

Newly transformed people, newbies, are suddenly no longer into these questionable pastimes and/or prejudices as are their (former) friends. That's what happens when they, the once normal folks, turn into health-conscious individuals who suddenly become justifiably aggravated with the cynics and all of their absurd chatter.

A newly transformed person quickly becomes wired differently. He becomes a whole different human. He no longer does the same things, feels the same way, or thinks the same as he once did. He then wonders about his recent past. How could he ever have downed all of that Mountain Dew? Or what was he ever thinking of with his twice-weekly reward bag of M & Ms (the economy size)?

It would be great if he critically went around questioning his other friends about why they still did this kid stuff (as we call these things, unlike the Normal Majority who thinks you can't do without them), but we care only that he is just now, perhaps for the very first time in forty-plus years, living like a health-conscious human being. This is what follows from the insight: "I *don't* have to be this way," which is actually the same as the unspoken but far more intelligent "Now I really *do* know."

This major turnabout is not the same for everyone. Some wake up one morning raring to go, getting completely into all of the right things. This is a very hopeful orientation, which we wish were true for all who make this sudden basic shift.

But others wake up scared that something very bad will happen if they don't start doing what they should. Perhaps whatever works is okay, but we wish these folks weren't quite as afflicted as they are. This is almost like getting that old doctor threat: "If you don't start doing something now, you might not be around for Christmas."

Anyway, some wake up painfully aware that if they neglect their bodies they will lose their shape. That is another way saying that they will go downhill (a Normal Majority fear that generally accompanies thoughts about dementia in old age) if they don't start doing something right now. All by itself, this causes profound anxiety, or at the very least, major stress.

However, in conjunction with "Well, I guess I'll start eating more fruits and vegetables and maybe do a weekly fast," this is not so bad, and almost good. It is reminiscent of: "Don't get rid of a bad habit until you have a good one to replace it with," the psychologists' battle cry back in the 1980s. No one really doubted the wisdom of that back then, nor do they today. Yet it doesn't get said often enough.

There still seems to be an all-pervasive chronic clinging to sugary pop, real food with its dangerous preservatives, chips with lots of bad fat, red meat, and endless R&R (along with porking out in Vegas, and drinking martinis to ease the pain of losing at the tables). This is even true of the folks who wake up knowing they have to change. They still fundamentally believe that the bad stuff is good for you, not like all the raw organic food which costs a lot and gives you diarrhea (so they believe). That's Health Nut stuff, and I'm not a one of those yet, I don't think.

Fortunately, there are still people who quietly demonstrate that the Good Life isn't just the way of all American flesh. Maybe that's a consolation to a new convert; maybe it will make them hang on. We hope so. There is a Jack LaLanne who knew from early on what you had to do, what would work and what wouldn't. More recently there is forty-two-year-old Olympic swimmer, Dara Torres, who literally gets better by the year and who has no intention of missing out on the competition in the next games four years out. Prior to her there was a Jane Fonda—or, there still is. She, too, looks far better than she is supposed to given her chronological age (the one on her driver's license). She did as much with her videos to help the women of the US in the 1970s as LaLanne did on TV in the late 1950s.

Most certainly, there are others hidden among the masses, it's just that we don't ever hear anything about them. E-mail us if one sits next to you in church, okay? But more to the point, where did these people's brilliance originally come from? Why and how were they so smart when so many others seemed to have arrogantly missed out with their "I didn't know"s?

We think that brilliance came to the superstars in an a priori fashion: it suddenly existed in the mind independent of experience. Some people just get smart like this, often at a very early age. It's as if they're educated one day by brilliant folks from outer space. They just get to know things that make them able to see when everyone else is blind. Their insight is more like a miracle from out of nowhere than a natural phenomenon—something that comes into being via discernible stages.

The trouble is that in our scientific age, we're not supposed to believe in miracles like this. In other words, it's the hallmark of maturity to believe only in natural progression. So maybe it's just a side effect of our scientific age that we have to go step by step in order for things to be real. Not really a bad thing, we're sure you'd agree. But we are suggesting an "A-ha!" experience of sorts as being responsible for the really outstanding individuals.

Anyone familiar with this pop term (coined by Fritz Perls), or the more formal a priori, will probably cringe at its usage in relation to athletics. A priori especially is generally associated with the high-minded intellectual pursuits of philosophy, theology, epistemology, and the like. In other words, you don't find it in relation to Health Nut–ology, which is not seen as a very important mental pursuit. This in itself may be the major cause of the problem.

Thinking you're above and beyond something makes contemplating it intolerable. It causes people to not think, not do, and not feel the way they should toward diet, supplementation, and exercise. Therefore, these topics supposedly ought not to be on a mature person's mind.

The situation is reminiscent of the way things were in high school toward phys ed. That class never had the clout of trigonometry or even social studies. Further, the male instructor was never the head coach of the football team. He was the JV, junior varsity, coach at best. The female instructor may have been head of the cheerleader squad, but no one ever took cheerleading very seriously, did they?

This is all problematic, as most of us use our bodies far more than our sine and cosine tables, or the population figures for Gary, Indiana. Nevertheless, that is the way it was fifty years ago, and it really isn't much different today. Physical conditioning just hasn't been a top priority. So why should anyone (in the Normal Majority, that is) have to know all that much about it? In this light, it seems "I didn't know" so proudly spoken makes sense.

Strangely enough, however, there is a glaring contradiction to this absence of knowledge, or arrogant ignorance. It comes in the form of the surefire cure of walking when dieting. This always works, as everyone is supposed to know, according to the Normal Majority. Cutting calories to below 1,500 when doing a daily half hour's worth of something as simple as walking (no club membership for fancy machines required) works every time. It is living proof that people eat too damn much and sit too many hours on their butts, as the Normal Majority knows. Everyone else over two, of course, is supposed to know this as well, even if they have never done it. Same goes for all of the fat kids in New Jersey who just appeared on CNN; they're just aren't applying themselves. (This is a sad phenomenon, we're sure you'd agree, given the problematic nature of the food they eat, its availability, and its relative low cost.)

The average adult of the Normal Majority will demonstrate these profound convictions when confronted by a friend or family member who is approaching obesity. He will then sonorously (and very deeply and profoundly) say, "If only you had cut your calories and done your walking, you wouldn't have this problem." But when it comes to himself, this obnoxious I-know-everything attitude never applies. He never practices what he is compelled to preach.

Everyone who knows that the 1,500-calorie-plus-walking plan will always work conveniently blocks this knowledge out when trying to get rid of their own Christmas cookie build up. It's as if they're living in denial over the basics. Apparently this is because worrying over a few trifles is not very grown-up. Other things in life, like who'll win the Rose Bowl, are far more important. Five extra pounds from a few good get-togethers are not curtains, not obesity. Besides, a little bit of extra (that bought-and-paid-for look) proves you aren't a kid anymore, which is supposedly good. It maybe even shows that you know how to live or proves you're not bankrupt.

According to the Normal Majority, those who are well-off can afford to eat more and take it easier than the not-yet-established folks who live in continuous anxiety. This doesn't really square with reports on low-income folks who very unfortunately tend to be the worst abusers of Mountain Dew and McDonald's filler-uppers, largely because they're cheap, in-your-face available, and tasty. Horrifyingly, the obesity epidemic pretty much starts at this point, irrespective of age.

But our concern here is more with the over forty-five, relatively well-off crowd who still feel the need to overdo it on Christmas cookies, frequent the Golden Arches every week, enjoy Buds with the game, and do all of the other self-destructive living that is so much a part of the American good life. Thus we ask, "What if this is the fourth time that you have done nothing to get back into shape after having overdone it since Thanksgiving?" Friends, that really shouldn't be. In other words, you should just cut back, and do it now.

The "I didn't know" crowd, in spite of everything, continues to tenaciously hang on to never having been enlightened. They stand firm on not having known anything when they could have taken a few simple Health Nut things seriously. Maybe there was a study that gave a flimsy reason why some Health Nutty thing just wasn't all it was cracked up to be. (There actually was a big grad school study some years ago that proved that exercise didn't necessarily make you healthier!) This enables them to hang onto the tried and true, as they call it: the FDA approval and the okay checkup from the doctor.

When it comes to vitamins, you hear people say they didn't know that all of our foods were really as nutritionless, as the natural foods people keep saying. The objection even goes further when they refuse to spend any extra money for organic foods just because some washed-out Health Nut thinks they should. Besides, "I dimly remember someone like that who burned the American flag back when she was in college."

When it comes to groceries, there also is the belief that red meat could really be that bad for you. I grew up on steaks and chops; everybody did, didn't they? So if they really are all that bad, why doesn't the FDA say something? This is the type of thing that goes on and on while the country gets fatter and increasingly more prone to dread diseases. It's "I didn't know"…"I didn't know"…"I didn't know," along with the tacit "So don't blame me for your and my physical trouble. Just get busy making us a cure in the form of a pill."

How can it be that there is such arrogant mindlessness? We think it's because the Big People's (the drug companies, the FDA, the local physicians, the media, wide-sided Congresspeople) propaganda is so good that it's taken as the gospel truth. The ads on TV are brilliant in their awful way. Furthermore, the anchorpeople aren't strange like the Health Nuts and they all look great. Surely they eat like you'd expect, wouldn't you think?

In our progressive, high-tech society, the big drug companies are almost always portrayed as the saviors from illness for the world. Okay, they make big profits, but they make astounding pills. The wonders of modern science are always played up, even when they cause thousands of problems, generating class-action suits. The conclusion apparently is that some of this kind of thing happens as society progresses, and they, the AMA, have ways of taking care of all that. No matter how serious a particular recall may have been, it's never as bad as the one high school kid in Kansas who overdid it on an athletic supplement. That, friends, is the epitome of having been brainwashed (or is it brain-dirtied).

What's never remembered is that the big people of the Normal Majority, the corporate giants and the politicians, are really most interested in making sure that the economy keeps on going and that Thanksgiving stays the way it has always been. Furthermore, the real people, the Normal Majority, their constituents, rather like things the way they are. So don't rock the boat, right?

All of these people want things to go on as they are so that the social fabric remains intact. Their implicit advice to all of the other real people (grown-up adults) like themselves is to stay away from the (childish) Health Nuts. That will keep the country safe and make you guiltless so you can sonorously recite your "I didn't know" whenever you might have to.

Poking fun at these folks or blaming them for their ignorance is futile. Besides, it might not even make good sense to do so. Ms. D and I are not so sure that any could really have known or acted any differently. They all may be hopelessly deluded. The Big People with their advertisements and news reports have really outdone themselves in making asses out of the masses. Were it not for the alternative folks (Health Nuts) we'd all be safe, so their message goes. Can anyone really use their head in the midst of this rhetorical din? The answer, of course, is yes, and it's essential that we all try; but the ability to do that will not come easily.

The latest lure for advertisers is to emphasize a genetic disorder as the primary cause for why you have a problem. If only your genes were different, then you wouldn't look or feel the way you do. Worse yet, if only your genes were different, you would get in great shape from just a little golf, watching what you eat, and staying away from the goodies. But that's not the best. Last but not least, if diet and exercise aren't enough, it's due to your genes from your great-aunt Jeanne. In other words, it's not at all because of your half-hearted efforts at the club. No way!

Helloooooooo! Friends, the drug companies are trying to get your money. That's why they're making it easy on you, letting you off the hook. Their free ride for you is something you really don't deserve. You do know this, don't you? Or do you really still think that trusting them is warranted by their FDA endorsements?

The quicker you start trusting your head more than you trust them, the better for you and everyone around you (like your kids, whom you influence without even trying). Buying into all of the drug companies' cheap grace is the very thing that will get us as a nation. It will lead to greater complacency, inactivity, idleness, and just plain sedentary living. What's more, it will make you unable to see the real causes of the forces that affect you.

The real question is "When are you going wake up with your 'A-ha' experience?" When will you realize that you are constantly being persuaded to live in a way that primarily promotes the Big People's livelihoods and political agendas, doing relatively less to make you healthier? But perhaps you vehemently disagree.

There are some who actually do not believe this: the "I didn't know" wing of the Normal Majority. These folks apparently just never see the articles on New Age healthiness, the longevity studies from a university, the ads for antioxidants, the endless e-mails promoting acai berries, or Jack LaLanne with the world's healthiest physique promoting his juicer. Or if these people have seen one or more of these things, they haven't taken any of them as seriously as the commercials for the new wonder pill (for pretty close to free maybe) from Astra Zeneca, or the R&R prescription from their doctor.

Friends, make your own turnaround today. Just stop buying into all of this American good life stuff and come over to the GOFHW program, the alternative that is really good for you in the long run.

Conclusion

Do think and educate yourself so you will experience your own "A-ha."
Don't leave your health in someone else's hands.

18

"Why Don't You?"
... "Yes, But"?

Have you ever shared a personal problem with a group of people? You *should* answer, "No, I would never do that" (unless it was in a therapy group run by a respected psychologist). But you will probably say, "Sure, hasn't everybody?" This is a common way of trying to prove that you are an okay person, a human being who is not perfect and who does not know everything. Everyone has done this at a party at least once, even the folks who try to come off as if they have all of the answers.

The expected result of sharing your weakness is that everyone present will like you more. You will prove that you do not live life on a pedestal and that others can therefore feel comfortable around you. In an addition, you may hear a worthwhile idea that is absolutely brand new. Or you may hear some unique point of view that will cause you to see the whole world differently. But this is highly unlikely.

Far more common is that you already know what everyone is going to say anyway, and that nothing they say can make a difference. So why would you even bother to go through the motions? You do so because part of you does not want to change. As has been implied elsewhere in these pages, change is hard on people, including you. Thus, if no one in your group comes up with anything earthshaking, you have every right to remain as you are, no matter how badly you may feel about it. Hearing nothing new reaffirms your conviction that your problem is hopeless and that you don't have to do anything about it except stoically bear it.

When it comes to exercise, problems always arise. They are as predictable as their ineffective solutions. One such problem is the inability to find enough hours in the day to squeeze in a workout. This is typical with those who have a long commute and/or a few young children. They say something like, "I know I should work out more, but I never have the energy after a whole day at work." Then some seemingly intelligent person responds "Why don't you just go the club every day before going to work?"

Of course, you have already thought of this. But getting up earlier means going to bed earlier, which is something you don't want to do, generally because it would cut into family time at best, or your favorite TV programs at worst.

We all know that with your family on your side, you could do this. You could be so energized by having their support that you might not even need that third cup of coffee in the morning. But gaining their allegiance is something you may not know how to pull off. A good head of the household *would* know, however, and that is what you are expected to be— either head of the house or revered first lady. But you aren't, and your inadequacy in this department is not something you want to bring up with a group of people.

So you say instead, "Yes, but then I won't have enough time to spend with the family." This makes you look like you know what you're doing as head of the house, that you are a model spouse and parent putting others' needs before your own. That will get you off the hook in the minds of most, including yourself (unless you are brutally honest in private, as you should be). As a result, sadly, it will become socially okay to continue to let yourself pear-shape out. You can then say, "I couldn't take time away from the family just to look good on the beach. After all, that is pretty high school, wouldn't you all agree?"

This might sound reasonable and even, I dare say, mature. Parents, husbands, and wives are expected to be beyond auditioning for *Baywatch*. Everyone, meaning all persons over forty-five, ought to know that by now, saith the Normal Majority. There are more important things in life than looking like a lifeguard or beach bunny. Mature, concerned, loving adults are expected to know this and to live their lives accordingly.

We have no problem with any of that. But what about cutting down on the costly prescription meds and eliminating the time off for expensive operations by just plain being optimally healthy? That in itself really can be a by-product of looking great for the beach. In fact, it will be, if you really go all out to absolutely look your best.

Yet not everyone sees it this way. If you're living healthily like doctor advises to ward off diabetes, it's pretty grim and that makes it okay. But if you're doing it to be in magazine photos, it's a whole different animal. Of course, Ms. D and I think that if you are into the latter early enough, you'll never have to worry about being into the former later on. But that's just us. In other words, we think that if you had committed to looking good on the beach for your Ponce or MsD when you first started going together, everything else would be falling into place right now.

But what we have is what we have, even if we always wonder why there was never an old adage like "A workout a day keeps the surgeon away." That would surely be more effective than the similar one with the proverbial apple (which never did have the amount of fiber you really need on a daily basis). So, anyway, you should just get with it, and we're sure that by now you most likely agree.

To other people who still don't think like this, the idea of an hour a day at the club for forty-five minutes of cycling and fifteen of lifting is just kids' stuff. It's seen as something that strokes your vanity, creating a conceited person more fit for flirting at the coffee shop than persuading others in the boardroom. It's not mature, not adultlike. It's not at all about being a real person. Thus it's something of which only a Health Nut is thought capable. Working out, supplementing, and eating right actually promote healthiness and maximum human effectiveness, i.e., real maturity, completely fanciful to the Normal Majority.

The same goes for the idea of getting healthier when you're already healthy. This one is *really* problematic! To the Normal Majority it's like fixing something when it ain't broken. According to them, adults should make far better use of their time by being part of the PTA, collecting the offering on Sunday morning, or being on the city council. All of these are more appropriate for people no longer on the make.

Their thinking is that no one should be wasting time dieting, working out, and supplementing anyway—unless, of course, it's part of their doctor's exercise program to ward off diabetes or some other troublesome illness. Nevertheless, even to these anti-cosmetic Normal Majority folks, it is considered prudent to watch what you eat, walk up a flight of steps or two instead of taking the elevator, and maybe take a One A Day. But that's hardly the same as trying to look enviable on the beach, they're sure we'd all agree!

Granted, they do allow you certain latitude in maintaining your appearance. Everyone is expected to do this for his self-esteem, the supposed beneficent brother of "ad boy/flaunting girl" pride. There is some good in this, so they think, but it's unclear what. Maybe it makes it okay to be seen with you in a restaurant or in a welcoming committee composite shot. Whatever, it is the acceptable opposite of letting yourself go. Yet going beyond the maintenance point gets you a "What are you trying to prove?" Plus there may be suspicions that you are looking for affairs, thereby ruining your chances of celebrating your twenty-fifth anniversary.

Back at the party, in a hall filled with people like this, your major objective is to prove that you're a likable, for-real adult—a good parent and faithful spouse. That's why you play the phony "Why don't you?" … "Yes, but" game. Everybody there should know that if you really wanted to live like a champion you'd be doing it and you would most *certainly* not be within ten miles of this insipid bushel of couch potatoes. But you don't. If you did, it would mean that you would have to confront your own mediocrity. No average person ever wants to do that! So you're safe. You can be as phony as you might like, or for as long as they're able to put up with you (or as long as you can stand it).

Saying that you can't fit exercise into your already impossible schedule is a way of convincingly saying that you are just as mature as everyone else at this pathetic party. It demonstrates that you are too busy with important things to be involved in looking bikini-perfect by July. This is similar to how Cheney came across when he and Bush first got into the White House. Bush was pictured out on the trail, running with his aides and Secret Service people twenty years his junior. On the other hand, Cheney was pictured poring over documents only to wind up in a hospital bed following a heart attack.

Now I ask you, which was the more mature statesman? I mean which one actually *was,* not which one *appeared* to be. Ms. D says, "Well, Bush, of course. He was wisely taking care of his health so he could do the best possible job." What she means is that she was sure that he would be the most capable of wisely pressing the button if necessary and of making relatively swift decisions on more than a few matters at once. In other words, he would be the most reliable one for the nonstop, fourteen-hours-per-day decision-making responsibilities of this country's leader.

To the average Normal Majority constituent, it didn't look that way. It looked like only Cheney could do well on the button issue, presumably relegating the other lesser matters, such as global warming, etc., to the left or right sides of the aisle. George W in shorts with the young guys just didn't cut it when it came to worrying about grown-up trouble.

Anyway, being a weighed-down adult gets you grown-up (old) points, otherwise known as respect. That's initially what Cheney got (thanks to the press portrayal), which is what forty-ish stockbrokers get when they act seriously and don't do anything to keep their hair from turning white or gray. (You might try mega-multivitamins if you don't want to follow suit.) Some, of course, purposely dye their hair white or grey like the ancient Athenian who thought that no one would ever believe wise words from a young mouth.

Meanwhile, back at the party, you should be sensing that all of the "Why don't you? … Yes, but" talk is getting phonier by the minute. People who play this game know the answers to their questions already. It's like their minds are already made up so they don't want to be confused with facts. Therefore, the whole back-and-forth exchange goes on like a superficially concerned polite conversation, which is boring on both sides but is more sincere on the parts of the people who are trying to help. Most often they are thoroughly bewildered that none of their suggestions are working.

Switching gears a bit, consider the early years of the battery-powered toothbrush, whiteners, and the like. Can you even for a moment think of someone at a party saying, "I think I'm going to get one of those new kinds of brushes like the dentist uses and buy some of that super-whitening toothpaste." Would anyone ever make an announcement like that? What do you think? Our guess is no, that would never happen. People just started using the new stuff and began dazzling their friends with an iridescent smile. So much for wasting breath at parties!

You would think working out would be the same, wouldn't you? Maybe in the next thirty years it will be. Right now, working out, supplementation, and diet are still in the marginal-to-crazy category. That's why the people who do them are called Health Nuts. What's worse is that they call themselves this as well. Doing that is bad, as it can eventually really make you not want to do what you should be doing; you just sort of pretend to be doing it, if you keep it up at all. Or you call yourself a Health Nut to keep all of your normal friends liking you. Then you are one down and able to accept everything that goes along with that.

Of course, we could be dead wrong about all of this. So let us know if you think we are. Maybe there is some good that will come of one of these helpful conversations. If you ever come up with anything that gets you into a gym or running around the block by sharing your problem with a bunch of couch potatoes, e-mail us or call, even if it's 2 a.m. That's not going to happen, and we think you know that.

In spite of this cynicism, we do believe that there really is a part of you that would like to be doing what you should. That's in spite of the fact that you just demonstrated your partial unwillingness to change. It's just that you don't know how to tap into the good part of yourself. So if you really would like to get into everyday workouts, here's how to pull it off. Just ask yourself over and over, in private: "Why *really* don't I start actually working out?"

At first you won't get much of an answer. But if you do it again and again while doing nothing else, you will. That's the key right there—you dialoguing with yourself, not someone else, and not with the radio blaring in the background. Then, and only then, the "I know I should, but" or "I haven't got time right now" won't be enough. That's the way it should be. Then you will have to come up with something far better. Eventually, you'll come up with the right answer.

Nevertheless, there is one drawback. *You may find that the real reason for your inertia is something you did not want to know about yourself.* But now that you do know it, you will have the power to change. Radical honesty, in private, pays off. That's the rainbow at the end of the storm. Oh, and there is a perk: you needn't e-mail us, or anyone else, with what you found out.

Conclusion

Do spend time alone asking tough questions.
Don't seek kudos form the Normal Majority.

19

Wearout-O-Phobia

Wearing out is the supposedly inevitable bad end of hard work. In other words, people think that if you work hard at anything physical, you are not just working hard or working intensely, you really are overdoing it. According to them, the unhappy result is that you will be unable to do even range-of-motion exercises when you get to the nursing home, assuming you are even lucky enough to make it there.

The reason the Normal Majority gives you for this is that exercise involves physical exertion, which becomes less and less possible as one gets older. That's because the cells start to die one day after birth, a few at a time presumably, but cascading horrendously as one gets older. Consequently, people end up looking the way they do in the nursing home, assuming they haven't more mercifully died in their sleep some years earlier. Thinking that this doesn't have to happen, that they could have turned back the clock with diet, supplementation, and exercise, is a fairy tale that only a Health Nut could take seriously.

Most people believe that we all get older-looking as we celebrate our birthdays, and that nothing can be done about it. Accepting one's loss of fitness is supposed to be part of growing old gracefully. Thinking otherwise is at best illusory (Health Nutty). One is expected to give up trying to look youthful when he's forty-five (vanity) or acting like he's still in high school training for the state meet. Those who don't or won't are given the scarlet letter of Health Nut. Even the peerless Jack LaLanne probably suffered from this stigma for decades.

As we've said elsewhere, Jack's philosophy has always been that the body gets better the more you work at it. This is the opposite of "Too many workouts shorten your life span," the standard belief of the Normal Majority. Of course, none of these authorities ever talks specifically about how many years it's supposed to cut off, or when you should start slowing down, or how slow "slow" is. Those things would require a lot of thinking about sports and health, something not all that important for mature living. All they know, therefore, is what they need to know, namely that overdoing it is not something you should let happen. That's why these normal folks all start one day after around age forty-five cutting way back so that they can begin planning for their sunset years.

It's the cutting back that is really supposed to be good for you. In fact, it's supposedly essential. The belief is that if you don't do it, you are asking for trouble. So slowing down is prudent and mandatory. In fact, starting earlier would not be the worst idea either. Wearout just happens, even if you do not burn out at your job. The energy for physical activities just goes away, and nothing can be done to stop it or replenish it.

The trouble with this is that LaLanne is still alive and exceptional in 2009 and there are older others who are also staying very well preserved for far longer than expected. So an increasing number today know that talk about wearing out is all mindless chatter. But they are statistically insignificant. The Normal Majority is still in the main and still in command with its supposedly well-intentioned advice and obnoxious criticism of those who dare to be different.

These self-righteous, ostensibly likable, allegedly well-intentioned folks are sneaky. They are like dirty bombs, only psychologically toxic instead of physically toxic, like those great-tasting Big Macs. They come across like people you cannot do without, friendly-like so that they can gradually wear you down one day at a time. They're only interested in saving you by helping you to see the folly of your ways. They are only trying to help you, which is what any good person would do for another, wouldn't you agree? That's why they do what you do, warmly smiling as they do it.

Speaking of Big Macs, the Normal Majority thinks that they're okay in moderation (like one instead of three per day). To them, they're harmlessly enjoyable. So why would Health Nuts like us have a problem with them? It's the quantity that does it, just like anything else. All things in moderation and you're safe. Besides, everyone ought to know that fun food now and then makes life worth living and won't cause any trouble. After all, Big Macs are FDA approved and the health inspectors don't ever shut the Golden Arch folks down. So they must be okay. Who in their right mind doesn't like a few of these with some fries and a malt? They're perfect picker-uppers when you're getting down from too much work, like a whole week of it at the office. To be perfectly honest, then, it's the job that gets you, not the gut bombs. So you can ignore what the Health Nuts preach—most of them don't have real jobs anyway! Don't you feel well taken care of now that you know all this?

This type of thinking makes us shudder at how unaware people can really be. A splurge like this, maybe a midweek picker-upper followed by a TGIF celebration, is disastrous over a six-month period of intense training. It's even worse within the context of the near-sedentary American good life. And our horror at it is hardly a new austerity. I've seen high school swim coaches buy those burgers and fries from their best freestylers and then throw them away in front of the whole team. Too, LaLanne has been on a similar kick ever since his first TV programs, which can still be seen on his website. In short, our supposed new aversion has been around for forty-five years—pretty much the same amount of time as the chronological age of the Normal Majority member, who's probably set to retire—the only reasonable relief after a life of being worn out by the job.

Friends, with gut bomb diets like these, it is easy to see why the Normal Majority fears wearing out. The amount of energy required to digest and carry them around is enough to burden anyone. We'd be tired out just like them if we followed suit, and we know you would be too, or have been. We just know the tiredness wouldn't come from the number of birthdays or from the numbers of rigorous daily workouts. Rather, it would come from decades of eating the wrong things, not working out, and staying away from supplements. Abusing yourself like that will make you tired, and it can result in a heart attack, to say nothing of a severely shortened lifespan.

Relentless, year after year strain on the heart is harder on a person than LaLanne pulling barges in San Francisco Bay. So in that context, we can definitely see where wearout-o-phobes are coming from. It's just that they blame their jobs instead of their living habits. What they do and don't do could have been (and should have been) different than it was!

You never hear good advice from the Normal Majority going something like "Better get off the couch and start acting like a college athlete." Even when it comes to their kids in their thirties, you seldom hear (seldom means one day out of 365, not one out of thirty-six) "Work hard" in place of a "Take it easy." Saying this to anyone other than an undisciplined adolescent would not only be rude, but also dangerous, so most people would think. The standard send-off here in the US now is "Have a nice day," which really means "Take it easy," as they used to say ten years ago. No normal person would ever think that a day of sweating and putting out could be even remotely nice. We're stuck in that old "Watch it, so you don't wear out" rut.

What would be a better thing to say? Personally, I wouldn't have a problem hearing or saying something like "Go for it." This is a variation of "Work hard," but "Work hard" suggests drudgery. "Go for it" suggests attaining your goal, which is more pleasant. You can even say this to someone in a wheelchair.

There are handicapped folks who really might like hearing it more than the standard "Have a great day." Some are excellent at sports like basketball and swimming. In a sense, these folks are in their own Jack LaLanne category. They are amazing in their own right. Refreshingly, they are not the norm. They have superlative attitudes in place of the Normal Majority's routine, conservative clichés, those of complacency, idleness, and ease. Apparently, these athletic individuals know nothing of the supposed inevitable bad ends of wearing out.

What you do find in the handicapped athlete is an acceptance of limitations alongside a surpassingly powerful will to overcome all obstacles. In other words, they say, "Yes, I have this problem" in the same breath as "No, I will never let it hold me back." What's needed is for the normal American to be like these folks with artificial limbs. Just as they say, "I do not have my flesh-and-blood legs anymore, but I won't let that hold me back," we all need to say, "Yes, I am no longer a high school kid," but "No, I will not allow this to keep me from having exceptional health." In other words, I would rather wear out training like I did in high school than rust out like all of my peers who are all going about acting their ages. We all have much to learn from disabled people.

Ms. D and I think it's really best for your own sense of survival to think like a high school athlete while keeping your mouth shut. But self-sacrificial Health Nuts could make a mission of talking about things like this. In a way, we'd love to see this even if we think it's too dangerous. Of course, health-conscious people believe in what they're up to along with being highly critical of what passes for grown-up common sense. They could put the Normal Majority in its place—one down, where it belongs. This might actually make us a better country after a while. That's exactly what the women did in the women's movement of the 1970s, winning recognition as real people deserving equal pay for equal work and equal respect for their contributions to their marriages and places of employment.

But we don't recommend that you follow suit. That's because the ladies had one advantage: there were overwhelmingly more of them than there are of you with your couple of new friends (the ones you have made by now, we hope). Further, you will have a big enough battle with yourself as you acquire new daily habits. You don't need another one with next door neighbors on either side, who are not going to approve of your efforts. So the best thing is just let them worry about you wearing out and get away from them as quickly as you can.

The over-forty-five Olympic hopefuls (older Health Nuts) need respect, especially when getting started. They need to have others off their backs so that they can maintain their workouts, supplementation, and diets. It's extraordinarily difficult to keep at these when you have lifelong friends from the Normal Majority who say they are on your side. Almost always, that makes it worse. Questions such as "How can I tell good old Frank that he's a mindlessly arrogant couch potato?" will plague you. After all, he was the one who helped you get the car out of the snowbank last winter. That's something you tend not to forget. The Normal Majority's putdowns, whether directly from the good old Franks or from the images of them you carry in your head, destroy diets, supplementation, and workouts.

There is no better explanation than this social-psychological one as to how there can be so much knowledge out there with so few people taking advantage of it. Everyone is afraid of what will be said about them for not taking care of themselves as they age (conserving energy so they don't wear out). Running every night before dinner is being a Health Nut, which causes the runners to hear anything from "An adult ought to care about important things" to "What's wrong with you that you cannot act your age?" No one wants to experience hearing such things because they imply that he is not doing what he should to take care of the life that God gave him. This even puts overdoing it into the seven deadly sins category, right alongside sloth and gluttony, if that's even remotely possible.

The only other reason to say that folks don't do what they should because they're afraid of the Normal Majority is that people are just lazy and unmotivated. That's what the Normal Majority thinks about anyone outside their circle. That's why they have such a profound faith in always having you consult with your MD before doing anything so risky as using your head about your own health. They are all convinced that you'll never make it on your own, as they surely could, of course, if only they were not too busy with mature living to try. You didn't know your good friends had such a low opinion of you, did you?

Trust me on this: even if your favorite Normal Majority person drives a '91 Chevy and you drive a brand new paid-off Beemer, he thinks he's better. That's what being the Normal

Majority is about. The same goes for his flabby waistline in relation to your washboard abs. They've been too busy working to have time for playing in the gym, or they've been spending time being a good wife and mother instead of frittering it away in the swimming pool. The quicker you realize this, the better.

If you take them seriously you'll find it harder to work out. If you don't get rid of them you will always feel uneasy because they will cause you to feel guilty and fearful of living like an athlete. And that, friends, is exactly what you must do to have more energy, whatever the age on your driver's license.

You must stay away from the Normal Majority with its fear of wearing out if you care about not being one of your health club's ninety-day statistics (wherein you start on 1/1 only to stop coming by 3/30). *The investment of energy produces more energy, and that is something they absolutely cannot comprehend.* They really think that hard work at this point in your life will cause bad things to happen. But that is precisely what you must do if you want to turn back the clock.

The norm for the Normal Majority is being ten to twenty pounds overweight, pessimistic about anything good coming from hard work, and angry at anyone who doesn't accept them and themselves just the way they are. ("I'm okay—you're okay," just like they said in the 1970s, remember?) This is a mature way of being, so they think, and so they expect you to think as well. Personally, Ms. D and I think this is arrogant—an all-knowing intellectual position based on insufficient facts and analysis, radically intolerant of anyone who would dare to disagree with them.

Friends, optimal health, also known in these pages as beach readiness, does not come from extreme makeovers or super genes as the Normal Majority believes. Rather, it comes from the far more mundane set of habits that get one labeled a Health Nut. These habits create energy, the exact opposite phenomenon that the Normal Majority fears the most.

The Normal Majority is so certain of inevitable wearout that it even hilariously cautions the physically fit, people who have been training for a number of years. These include their peers and even people like us, which makes it even more laughable.

Older athletes are appearing more on the covers of magazines than they ever did before, and that is good. But they still don't have the same clout as the heavyweight boxing champ or the 250-pound tackle in presumably okay tights who just scored the greatest number of touchdowns. The ones who stick in the imagination are the big boys, the guys who burn out right after hanging it up for the last season. These are the real heroes. The other folks are just super Health Nuts running around the block in shorts courting premature entry into the nursing home. Friends, for the good of the country, this kind of thinking has to stop.

Recently, the USA got a pretty good start at changing things with the coverage of the 2008 Olympic Games. Dara Torres got her place in the spotlight for a month or so. And she made it clear that she'd be back in 2012. No retirement for her, and no prediction of her imminent demise. She looks fantastic—in her own way as awesome as the great Jack LaLanne.

More of this has to happen (without eclipsing the much-younger Michael Phelps, who did a superlative job as well). There have to be a lot more Dara stories, and hopefully a few Daniel stories (a still-mythical forty-four-year-old male freestyle gold medal counterpart for Dara) as well. But it seems that we are talking about decades instead of months. Already, the glow of Dara in the summer has been eclipsed by the upcoming World Series, which will be followed by the Rose Bowl (both with real athletes in them, you see).

It's hard for a society to change its heroes, but that is what we as a nation must do. It's far easier for you personally and individually to choose whom you will focus upon. Choose the right ones and you'll lose your fear of wearing out early. You'll look forward to better years yet to come. Need we say more?

Conclusion

Do better today than you did yesterday.
Don't fear the consequences of hard work.

20

The First Ninety Days

Ms. D and I shouldn't feel badly about criticizing anyone in the interests of a fit America, but we do nonetheless. That's true especially of trainers in health clubs, underpaid as they are, overpaid as they're perceived as being. That's because we know that where they are coming from is heavily impacted by the big people: the AMA (today's answer to the Leon Medical Association of the sixteenth century), even a bigger influence than the doctors. Personal trainers know that if they don't adhere to AMA rules, which reduce to "Better safe than sorry," they will be fired and possibly sued.

You cannot be a certified trainer unless you go through the required schooling and adhere to the Normal Majority's rules of healthiness, also known as common sense. The assumption is that whatever the AMA teaches is what everybody should know anyway, unless we're talking about specific illnesses (kidney failure, diabetes, etc.) and methods for treating them. Therefore, the personal trainer's first obligation is to be like everyone else in the big gun Normal Majority (the AMA), committed to keeping anyone wanting to be healthy out of harm's way.

No one should really have a problem with this. Even a highly respected Olympic coach wouldn't think that one who had done nothing for the last twenty years should start off the day by swimming a mile every morning. No one would. But a good coach would wonder why he didn't if he had been building up to it for the last eighteen months. His present efforts should have ensured that something like that would eventually occur. If that were to happen, the world's newbies would have entirely different first-ninety-days periods.

That's our problem. Standard training routines never get off the ground the way they should. If only they were told to:

- ❖ Gradually increase resistance and rpms, while showing up consistently after having dieted and supplemented
- ❖ Get psyched up for a whole new lifestyle before even starting
- ❖ Keep making entries into a personal log
- ❖ Do one more rep this week than last
- ❖ Lengthen out that stride
- ❖ Pull harder in the water

If newbies had this advice and took it, they would benefit from a trainer and their first ninety days would be no problem at all.

Instead, the standard get-go, followed by nothing more than a little supervision by a personal trainer/membership counselor with clipboard in hand, goes something like this: "Do a few laps around the track three or four times a week, maybe along with a few of the machines, and work at cutting down on the goodies." That's it. It's the same thing your mom could have told you. But you got it from a trainer, so it must be good, right? Hopefully.

This may not be much, but it is better than nothing at all. Yes, friends, we'll take whatever we can get. If it won't hurtya, it just might help ya. It is the standard way to begin healthiness, American-style. And we're a little bit excited because you may, yes you *may*, have a one in fifty chance of making it past the first ninety days, and that really is more than zero in fifty!

Every trainer will suggest something like this for virtually anyone except the obviously infirm. That's mostly because it will not do any harm whatsoever and may actually allow nature to do a little good. Besides, it helps to keep you coming to the club, so maybe your trial membership will turn into a real one. As I've said before, trainers wear the membership counselor hat as well.

Ms. D and I think that this is like prescribing a One A Day low-dose vitamin to make someone get a little bit healthier over time. Anyone can do this. You will never hear anyone say, "Ask your doctor if a OneA Day now and then is right for you." That should tell you they're okay, or possibly ineffective. It should also make you have the good sense to compare the ingredient dosages with megadose multivitamins, which are OTCs (over the counter pills) as well. Anyway, they're presumably as safe as Tylenol, which is safer than aspirin nowadays. So let's leave it at that. The point is that they fall into the watered-down category along with all the other weak advice.

Of course, we don't think One A Days or any type of namby pamby support will help much, but that's mostly because we are concerned with people in consistent rigorous training (like the type we think you should be in). We know of heavy vitamin and mineral dosages that have been taken by athletes who wouldn't think of being without them. Not only do they know that their diets are not as nourishing as they could be, as a result of what's done to the food nowadays, but also that they are continually putting a lot of strain on their muscles and ligaments. This causes them to wear down, and they must therefore be refueled. Also, people who train know that the amount they might have to consume to get everything they need would have them eating all day—something that's not at all good for anyone! Most of this is common knowledge found on the Internet and in sports publications.

Nevertheless, the trainers will feel compelled to prescribe these boringly safe One A Day pills and programs to all the new people wanting to be healthier than they currently are. Yet maybe we shouldn't be too critical. The MDs won't prescribe any vitamins or workouts at all. And, as we've said before, something is better than nothing. This is true as long as you don't think weak substitutes are going to do something and wonder afterward why what you're doing isn't working.

So let's get back to your first attempt at getting off the ground with a personal trainer. Is this patronizing "Why not try a One A Day if you must" anything that someone starting out really wants to hear? No. What this sounds like is a never, never plan, one the newbie knows won't work anyway. It's just like everything else newbies have heard from Mom, Dad, and others all their lives. Granted, it may be a safely acceptable way to get off the ground, but, said in the usual tired way, it will be a turn-off when a new person can stand that least.

On the other hand, committed personal trainers who know what they're doing know that the One A Day stuff just isn't enough. But they won't tell you *that* either. Maybe you'd think they were Health Nuts if they did. Or worse, if you had a bad physical reaction such as a harmless niacin flush or some achy muscles, it might come back on them. So they're not inclined to be very aggressive. That leaves you pretty much on your own in this highly critical area that you may know very little about. And this is enough to make some newbies think about not showing up for workout number two.

But if you're the newbie who's still hanging in there, you are still hoping that your personal trainer can help you make something happen. You want what you want—to look good this summer on the beach, proud that your willpower has conquered all. As a result, you encourage him or her to dive right into the basics to help you, believing that this is the year you're finally going to get in shape for good. But that belief doesn't last for long.

You see no physical changes for the first four full weeks (oh my!), which leaves you feeling completely discouraged. It may lead to a newfound faith in something you know next to nothing about—genetics. Everybody knows everything about it nowadays. So you, an English major with a minor in business, start thinking that your genes just aren't the type that respond well to diet, exercise, and supplementation. That gives you good reason to quit on or about February 1, well within three months of your start on January 2.

Most likely, personal trainers won't question your thoughts or motives and will allow you to do just that—quit. You are the boss, the club member, and that's your right. From your perspective, you just wasted $20 per hour times three sessions per week for four weeks. From the personal trainers' perspective, they did everything they were supposed to do so your failure is just unfortunate. It happens most of the time, so they rather expected it anyway.

Of course, their opinions wouldn't have affected you, would they? That is, if they thought you were probably going to bomb out, that wouldn't have impacted any of the ways that they interrelated with you, right? Anyway, we're now onto same song, second verse—you have once again stopped the music.

After the quitting, there is boredom. You are now back to normal: no more turning into model material like you've seen in the Bowflex ads. You've simply had it. Things aren't going fast enough, so you've started to wonder if it might not have been easier to just say no to all of the second helpings, high-calorie cookies, and midnight snacks. If only you had just cut back on all of the goodies long ago, all would have fallen into line, right? The answer of course is yes, but that won't help in the least. You will be back to what feels right almost immediately. This results in the grown-up, sensible (non–Health Nut) decision that the energy invested in getting fit cannot be justified on the basis of the results: the reward does not justify the risk.

At this point you have either given up completely or finally confessed that you simply cannot do it on your own. For the first group, we have no time. They haven't done one ten-thousandth enough. With the second group, we are empathetic. Feeling like a failure is painful. After all, coming to your senses, you know now that you weren't at it for long enough and that you colluded with your lesser self by hanging it up way too early. You did not do what you ought to have done. You simply have to say, "Maybe I just don't have what it takes, which isn't good, because I know of others who do." That's very, very difficult, to put it mildly.

If you are a strong believer in self-determination, we commend you for your admission, which we know wasn't easy. You've bottomed out, so to speak. Things are bad; they can't get any worse. There is no will to go further. There is only self-doubt. Of course, we don't think it is all that bad, but we respect that admission. So bask in the good vibes of our positive regard, as long as you don't think that you just aren't a working-out type person like Ponce and Ms. D, perhaps.

Friends, there is no such individual. God made you able to move. *Period*. You just have to stick to it, that is, train yourself to be better at it, that's all. And that requires some internal decision work. You may now think that reaching out again is better than reaching in.

We are now talking about you shopping for a new personal trainer, probably at a different club. But this is like going from the Teflon frying pan into the iron one. In other words, you will not make much of an improvement. Neither of them, not the first or the second, will help much, and this is what you need to know. Being too aggressive could get a trainer sued or fired. That's why they are all pretty much same.

This one, like the last one, won't hurt you, and at the very least will be there when you show up. That is a good thing, as it may actually get you there when you might otherwise have been too adult-busy or whatever. With a little luck, you will realize that things are neither better nor worse so you might just as well hang in there and see where it takes you. This is the same as accepting your new trainer, which, if not optimal, is better than nothing. At least you will show up on a regular basis.

The only partial problem with this is that very few trainers have had the advantage of starting from the bottom of nowhereville, where you are starting from today. Most are simply fortunate to have come from good homes where there were good diets and where going out for a few sports in high school was encouraged. In other words, they are not really like Burgess Meredith in *Rocky Part I*.

Most of the personal trainers in the health clubs do not know how to build an athlete from the bottom up. Most of them are little more than boy-meets-girl attractive, which is way they were offered the job in the first place.

None of that is bad, to be sure. But it won't give them the confidence to kick you in the tail when you need it. At best they'll come up with something like "Listen to your body" or "Keep up the good work." Both of those sound good, but they seldom get said at the right time or for the right reasons. "Listen to your body" comes up when a workout starts to get a little tough (after a whole week of doing it) and "Keep up the good work" follows a lot of uninspired going through the motions. These both translate into "It's almost ten minutes until the end of this session, and this person probably won't be back tomorrow anyhow, thank God!"

What you need to hear from a trainer is "Stop feeling sorry for yourself and get on with working out." Burgess Meredith would say this to you, just like he did to Rocky. So if you have a Burgess clone, you're fortunate. But generally you won't, which means you won't hear what you need to hear. That's largely because, as we've said, standard personal trainers don't really know where you're at. They have been doing the right things since relatively early on and thus have at best forgotten what it's like to start out.

When you begin, it will be an uphill battle to just make it to the club. You will have more energy lags than you ever dreamed possible. Most personal trainers won't even really know how tough these are on you when they happen. Nor will they realize that they are making you feel like you're too old to be starting out. After all, you are over forty-five, so that's what the Normal Majority will tell you. And the trainers who are part of the pre-thirty-something crowd can't possibly know from experience how to get you through this.

Now, do we really have a problem with that? Well, we can forgive and understand, but you bet we have a problem! Everything we're telling you can be reduced to working out with the same regularity as brushing your teeth. You would never think of stopping your toothbrush routine after ninety days, right? No way! You'd do it every day, maybe twice a day, and use all of the best toothpastes. That's how you have to be in relation to your workouts, and it's a trainer's real job to get you there, whether you are thirty-two or sixty-two.

Therefore, what trainers need to say is, "I am glad you think I can help you, but unless you and I start agreeing on some things right now, by March you will have quit like almost everyone else. So first off, can you afford me for that long, and second, what do you think about what I just said?"

In short, they should get you to commit to not missing. That takes some personal clout, but what they're teaching is about as much of a no-brainer as knowing that you'll always have a great smile if you never miss your twice-daily toothbrushing routine. So you know what you want, and he or she knows what you have to do to make it happen. Simple, right? It is … *it really is.*

Nevertheless, keeping you on track won't be easy. That's why we don't trust anything short of a dedicated professional, also known as a coach. The standard personal trainer does not have that kind of authority.

What has to happen is pretty uncomplicated. You have to get beyond the first three months of the first year. Then you should be able to do it on your own until you have two years under your belt. That is 365 times two workouts (or 730 workouts), which is a lot of effort: hard work in relation to an extreme makeover, the quick fix as seen on TV.

That may sound grim, but it really isn't that bad. By the end of the twenty-fourth month, you will be as into your daily routine as the trainer is. (In fact, after the first 120 days, it will start to be fun.) That is the foremost reason for doing it the hard way instead of via the transformation as seen on the TV. Once you have the training spirit in you, you'll never go back to being a couch potato. In other words, GOFHW will actually prove superior to new technology and plastic surgery. You simply won't be tempted to go back to your bad old ways, and you won't be able to see how your friends can stay addicted to them (if you are even still talking to those people).

Friends, if you really need someone to help you get started, get a *real* trainer. Get someone like Burgess whom you really can call "Coach." They are tough to find, but they are out there. And not all of the others out there are as bad as I have made most out to be, to be sure. Some really aren't thinking about this weekend's date, or obsessed with the allegedly universal problem of a novice overdoing it. Some really may even have a useful tip or two on more than just the use of the equipment at the club.

Conclusion

Do make it through day ninety-one.
Don't be pacified by the One A Day approach.

21

The Not-So-Extreme Makeover

There is a TV show that combines everything needed to turn frogs into princes and goose girls into princesses. It includes, but is probably not limited to, plastic surgery, liposuction, weight training, dieting, juicing, hair styling and wardrobe counseling. These transformations are remarkable, but we wonder how many of them are permanent.

Admittedly, this book is about doing the same type of thing, but it's going to take two to three years. *Period!* Granted, we aren't up on hairstyle and fashion, but in that amount of time, we expect that you will be. *If* you do an adequate daily workout routine, eat a low-fat, low-carb diet, and supplement effectively, that will happen. Because you'll feel better about yourself, you will become more fashion conscious.

So why listen to us when you can get the same result or better in a much shorter period of time? After all, faster is always better, isn't it? Here are a few good reasons:

❖ Reason number one is that a commercial extreme makeover is cost prohibitive. The makeovers on TV are in the $30 to 40 K range, and they're not covered by insurance.

❖ Reason number two is that you must maintain the effects of the extreme makeover once you have had it. That can be almost impossible if you have never done anything to stay in shape and you just happened to go from a 3 to a 9.7 on the on-the-make scale. They don't tell you that, but you should at least suspect it.

A bodily makeover, with the exception of bone work, is hardly permanent. The new body is not going to stick around after crash dieting, supplementation, and some secret form of muscle blasting unless you treat it the way it needs to be treated. Even then there is some question as to how long it will remain if you haven't done any disciplined work prior to all of the cosmetic surgery. Maintaining an attractive body requires ongoing conditioning, not merely a one-time break from bad old habits only to see them again become dominant.

The fantasy is that once the surgeons do their work, you are changed forever. That really is pretty much like the standard Fountain of Youth mythology, wherein you take one drink of fountain water to turn back the clock forever. Ideally, that gets you back to your ideal appearance. That's how the fairy tale goes, and that's substantially the goal the makeover team is aiming for.

However, the whole truth is that the extreme makeover doesn't really give you a second chance for very long unless you stay with the proper diet, supplementation, and exercise: the catch that they never talk about. What it does is to realign some bones, take out some fat, change some of your body chemistry (for a short while at least), pump some muscles, and get you glamorous as you go through the wardrobe update as well. Then you walk into a room where everyone knows you and none of them can believe their eyes.

That's all great as long as you don't return to couch potato living, start regularly rewarding yourself with McDonald's. But you will go back to the same old tried and true if you do not work very hard at preventing it. You will return to the old you unless you really change internally. That is what you *must* do and it is not easy.

All of the hoops the medical team makes you jump through are like going to Army boot camp, where your drill sergeant turns you into a ninety-day wonder. You get in great shape along with all of the other recruits. But as soon as you are discharged, you go right back to the same old habits and the same old body. The completely flat stomach reverts to a spare tire and you return to puffing after one flight of stairs.

Sadly, the one-time recruits may even reminisce about this wondrous time years later, never having done a push-up during the interim. Of course, they don't look as hot now that they are civilians. The only ones who don't go back to normal are the drill sergeants, who continue to get better over the years. They of course have been at their jobs, in their Smokey the Bear hats, for at least ten years. Being like them, minus the ground-glass-for-breakfast demeanor, will do what you want and make us proud.

After watching the extreme makeover show for the first few times, Ms. D and I thought there must be some good in it that we were just plain missing. Unfortunately, we just couldn't really see it, but we knew how delighted everyone on the show became. Something that makes so many people so happy must have something wonderful about it. So we did some more thinking.

We pondered the possibility that an extreme makeover could give you a new start, something you could build from. In other words, it could cut off years of work, getting you out of the hole and up onto high ground, so to speak. Then you could go about doing the basics of workout, diet, and supplementation without having to do the initial eliminating of the abuses of the past. That's what we originally thought. But was this realistic?

Let's first assume that the surgeons can really transform a body structurally. (They do bone and oral surgery, so maybe there's a chance.) And let's say that they can take out tens of pounds of sheer fat, tuck up the saggy skin, and offer scar-free liposuction. And let's say they can do it well enough for the makeup artists to then work their magic.

But what happens afterward? Let's start with the psychological trauma of now being a size 6 when you have been accustomed to decades of living in the world as a 14. Trust me, not all of your friends will continue to be delighted in the change (the way they are on the TV show), and that will be upsetting. In fact, not one of them will be supportive for very long, unless they themselves are model-like. But even then, the competition would cause trouble. Therefore, the pressure on you to return to old habits (your former old self) will be irresistible. Here, more than any place other in this book, is where you need new friends.

Nevertheless, resisting is precisely what you must do, and there is strength in numbers. Thus you might actually make it by reaching out—with a lot of help from some new friends. But it will still not be easy, as you aren't thinking of moving to another state, we'll bet. Let's say you aren't.

In that case, you should get a crash course on what it means to be a champion, with the intent of internalizing it and never deviating from it. If you have no idea what it takes to get to the point where you currently are, you have some hard truths to swallow. You will have to acquire new habits so that your new body does not go away. Getting a book by an Olympic medal winner is a good place to start. Memorizing it is *not* a waste of time, nor is listening to the audio tapes at least ten times if some came with it.

Frankly, you might do well to find a hypnotist who knows what to program into you given what you are trying to pull off. Not just any hypnotist will do. You have to have one who can get to know you extremely well—who can learn what triggers your deviations from the norm, what makes you lean back when you really need to press forward, what makes you pig out when you should really fast, what makes you spend your money on something mature when you should have augmented your standard dose of vitamins, and the like.

This person probably doesn't exist, nor would even a very good one be willing to take enough time to get familiar with you unless you spent a lot of money with him or her. Even then, you would still have no real assurance that they would integrate all of the data correctly to program you appropriately. That's why we think it's most prudent to think it through on your own. Yet trying very hard to find close to the ideal may put you in touch with some very important things about yourself. Do any or all of this *before* you go for surgery, not after, and you really might have a chance.

You've got to let the voices of champions get into your head and you have to do what they say. They are supposed to drown out the voices of the Normal Majority and all of the media folks who caution you against overdoing, taking on too much too fast, saving your money on supplements that you only pee away anyway, etc. But if you find that you are still arguing with them and losing, you have to do something about it. Find a way for the new you to win the debate. In other words, you are going to have to really t.h.i.n.k. That may not be easy but it's better than quitting, only to start all over again at some distant time in the future.

When the going gets tough, you have to get going. When it feels like you can't do it, you have to work harder. When your jeans still look bad after a few weeks of work, you aren't putting enough into your workouts. Those are the types of things that need to be echoing in your brain, not "I'm not sure if this is right for me" or possibly "It may be that I'm just not an exercising type person," like they said in the 1970s. Those are the justifications for just showing up at the club and walking around the track a little when you've got the time. That's all part of the "I have to watch it at forty-five because I'm not thirty-five anymore" syndrome. Those are the truths (vital lies) that will get you.

Friends, you cannot just go through the motions expecting to turn into a champion. No champion ever was like this. If you've seen the original *Rocky* movie, you know what I mean. If you haven't seen it, see it a couple of times, whether you are a man or a woman. Then you'll know what it takes. Rocky has powerful voices in his head along with an incredible trainer in Burgess Meredith. And he has Adrian as his MsD! That's what you need if you are going to make it.

Champions go for the gold even before they start. They don't wait to see if they can win a few minor victories before they really get serious. If you are starting out at forty-five to do what you should have been doing since high school, you may be at a disadvantage. But that doesn't mean you can't make it. You just have to work harder. You simply must refuse to let this hold you back. That's what you absolutely must do.

Doing that requires more than just trying. That's why you need a former Olympic champion on tape for your headset. These people have been going for it—the gold, that is—since *before* their first workout. Just listening to his or her enthusiasm will pick you up better than a quart of coffee or two green tea caps. Then you really will get to the gym every day, probably at the same time or earlier, to do the same routine over and over again. And you will do it with more power and energy than you ever would have after listening to your friends in the Normal Majority with their words of caution they call wisdom.

Your future is in your hands. Just trade in their trite slogans like "Have a nice day" for your new friends' "Work on that stride." Then see what you look like in two to three years. We bet it really will be better than if you continue on with the tried-and-true good life of the couch potato thing. Trust that; skip the "Been there, done that" folks who are out to discourage you; hang in there past the first ninety days; and then just see what you think. What better do you have to do with this relatively small part of your life than what you must to make it longer and infinitely more enjoyable?

Anyway, that's *our* not so extreme makeover, which we have more faith in than the one on TV.

Conclusion

Do go after your permanent transformation.
Don't expect it in less than two years.

22
Epilogue

There is really not much else to say. If you want to look good on the beach, just go for it. Don't wonder if it's going to work. You need only to work out, supplement, and diet properly for a long enough period of time—two to three years and that will do it. That of course assumes you don't drink alcohol, smoke, or use drugs, which we haven't really talked about. We assume you don't do any of the bad things.

Maybe you do, however. If so, I seriously doubt whether any of the preceding has a chance of working. So drop the bad habits. That's step one, and if takes a while, it takes a while. Then listen to what we have to say again. Everything we are recommending is dependent upon having a physical constitution that is free from the hard stuff. The soft is bad enough (meaning anything from unfiltered water to Mountain Dew and dollar burgers). It is addictive in its own way.

We could have talked to anyone of any age, really. For the most part, though, we were concerned with baby boomers, like ourselves, starting with Dara Torres in her forties and working up to LaLanne at ninety-five. This is the generation that supposedly really cares about de-aging, living forever, and looking like movie stars, even though the Normal Majority thinks they can't—being over the hill, and all. That's the bland side of what the sensible folks, the Normal Majority, have to say.

The more colorful side is that people (you in particular, right here and now) ought to be concerned with more important things, which reduces to winding up your career and retiring from active citizenship. The Normal Majority thinks you should do that, becoming a grand and glorious senior citizen. They want you to study that AARP website and play by the rules.

Okay, that may be sensible, but we think this is the quickest way to rust out, turning into a prime candidate for a nursing home twenty years down the road. We know you don't want this, but what you *do* want may be too scary for you to articulate. The Normal Majority might overhear ("I heard that …," as they're fond of saying) and call you a Health Nut.

What most of these normal folks do not believe in is that you can turn back the clock.

Doing so is what the sixteenth-century Ponce DeLeon mythology was supposedly all about, and your grade school teacher told you how nuts he was. Yet that has never meant substituting numbers on your driver's license, and scientists are working on making people biologically younger as you read. Rather, getting younger really means catalyzing cell growth so that you can start losing the wrinkles, gray hair, negative attitudes, worn out body, and pot belly. These things generally separate the young from the old, and they are attainable for seasoned adults.

We think the USA is a sedentary culture, fostering premature aging by encouraging R&R. This is the American good life. Our position is that it is neither good nor American. It makes you saggy and unhealthy; therefore, it's bad. It is the result of the media and large company influences that inundate you with one-sided rhetoric (propaganda). Thus it is counter to our spirit of freedom, making it decidedly un-American.

People in our country feel the plight of obesity. This is a primary cause of other dread diseases that cost dearly in lives and dollars. It's been called an epidemic by the media. People do whatever they can to keep from catching it, right? Well, we don't think they do enough. This is evidenced by typical New Year's resolutions to lose the excess weight; after the first ninety days, most people are no longer doing it. We believe that's because of being pulled back by their friends, relatives, and neighbors, whom we have called the Normal Majority. We think these folks, well-meaning as they think they are, create incredible inertia on those who dare to be younger than their chronological age.

Problems happen right here in our homes when we dare to make this happen by starting to live a health-conscious life. It would be wonderful if husbands and wives could decide together on changing their living habits and never turn back. But it's all too often the case that one decides to do it and experiences the other's continued resistance. We have called this the wet blanket phenomenon. The belief is that beauty or attractiveness is more than skin deep and that it shouldn't be an issue in a healthy marriage. No one can take issue with that, except those who care about seeing a healthier America, a trimmer looking Main Street, USA, and maybe, just maybe, a more attractive person for their spouse.

Icons whom we have mentioned include Dara Torres, Jane Fonda, and Jack LaLanne. There are others too (Schwarzenegger, Stallone, etc.) but the first three initially come to mind. They have done much for our country, but why can't they be trainer generals, our joint chiefs of staff? Maybe it's because we haven't persuaded Congress to give them all titles. Who knows? This may sound facetious until you consider the hope of getting the USA into a preventative health mode instead of one that's concerned only with keeping us all okay.

Every day, people who aspire to be healthy do things that get them into trouble with the Normal Majority. The one big thing they do is to simply live healthily, supplementing, dieting, and working out all of the time, just like brushing their teeth, even on Christmas Day. Things like this earn them the Health Nut label. We think this has to go, just like the term "girl" went away because of women's liberation. Though we believe that it's hard enough getting people to the health club on a regular basis, health-conscious person's liberation has to happen or people will continue to feel one down for doing the things that have the greatest chance of reducing this country's astronomical health care costs! We hope that someone will pick up the banner and win the battle.

We treat our pets better in the US than we treat ourselves. We'd never share a morning donut and cup of coffee with

Barney the Beagle. And we absolutely would *never* grind up a cigarette to be put in his dish. Yet—need we say more? Barney gets dog food to be sure, and we get people food. The big trouble is that this generally means very healthy Alpo for him and cheeseburgers (non-organic stuff) for us.

No one can break away from the humdrum habits of this country without having some new friends. These are good people who don't look at you funny when you say no to Christmas cookies and yes to the rush that comes from today's workout, which was better than yesterday's. These choices get the standard person (Health Nut) into trouble with Normal Majority. There is only one defense against this deplorable situation and that is to get a support group. There is great strength in numbers.

Many today want more than merely aging right on schedule, which they know will come from living normally. That's why they take us seriously. We are all about GOFHW, and we really think it is good for everyone. Yet there are those who raise their eyebrows and caution the gullible ones who might be led down the garden path by Health Nutty people like us. These concerned folks may have seen numerous people fall apart by pushing out in the swimming pool, more than one death from anorexia, or countless severe problems that have been the result of herbal overdose. But we rather doubt it.

There is such resistance to the concept of hard work that we have been compelled to give examples of how it has caused miracles. We know this seems fanciful to the modern-day way of thinking, where plastic surgery and steroids seem to make the only real overnight differences, but we have seen the same happen after consistent hard work. The only way GOFHW makes sense is to think of water trickling down a hillside. If it's done long enough without stopping, it creates a river.

The Normal Majority thinks Ms. D and I are too severe for our own good. They think we should stand in front of our barn with a pitchfork just like the subjects in *American Gothic*. That's fine. The imagery isn't all that appealing to us either. But we just think it's time to stop all of the easy answers with the latest drug from Pfizer, which addresses your health problems on the basis of your genes. Maybe you really do have a problem that is gene-based but, friends, be honest: are you really putting out all of your energy on the bike at the club, or are you talking on the cell phone?

Older people are getting more and more into diet, supplementation, and exercise. We're not really sure why, but we know they are. Maybe LaLanne is their inspiration? Possibly, but probably not. Even these sixty-five-plus folks can't really relate to such a peerless wonder. Yet many are vegetable juicing everyday and not stopping until they've walked for an hour around the mall. Jack is supportive of all of that, to be sure. So are we. We'd like to see younger generations doing this as well.

Ms. D and I think that the sixty-five-plus crowd simply has an easier time sticking to what they started out doing, excelling at it. Sounds a whole lot like GOFHW, doesn't it? That's just part of being older, possibly. In addition, they're retired, with hours during the day that younger folks don't have. Anyway, they can be seen walking a lot and lifting weights. And studies have shown cellular changes to have occurred in *fewer than six months!* The implications are staggering for everyone. If only we'd all start taking things like this seriously!

In our judgment, there is only one sure way to make it only to seventy-five, when you could have made it to 145. That is to just lean back and take all those little signs of aging seriously (growing old gracefully, aging right on schedule), seeing the handwriting on the wall when you feel really tired after yesterday's run. That's part and parcel of the life of ease (those hazy crazy days of soda, and pretzels, and beer), which is pretty much drug-like in itself. The Normal Majority makes a huge deal out of all of that. They think you should too. After all, what would the Fourth of July be like if you and everyone else didn't get all wow, whoopee over the same old stuff? But maybe you don't care, and maybe, just maybe, we've got you started on the road to a healthier, more vibrant, more attractive, and more fit you.

If so, and if you started doing something today (please tell us you already did), let us know how you figured out how much exercising you should be doing. There are numerous ways to determine this, assuming you actually make the big dive into working out to begin with. We have recommended the seek-and-ye-shall-find approach, experimenting with different resistances and asking yourself if you can do the same again tomorrow. This is the best one for a person who still has the brain God gave him or her. But we know the Normal Majority prefers having you think that these are only things that your doctor should advise you on even if he or she would never make it to the pool before doing morning rounds at the hospital.

Friends, you can go for help on the whole megahealth issue if you'd like. You can have *the conversation* with your doctor; you can get an expensive trainer like Oprah's; you can get someone with a clipboard to show you the ropes; and you can sign up for plastic surgery and wardrobe consulting. You can even ask your out-of-shape friends what they think in hopes of getting inspired by folks who know little more than "You oughta be taking it easy if you're gettin' up there like all of us." Who knows? After all, wisdom cries out in the streets, right?

You can do any and all of these, or you can take us seriously. We've made a strong case for the latter. But you are the one who must finally decide whom you will listen to. Ms. D and I, of course, hope that you opt for your own inner voice. But all we can really do is wish you the best in the process.

Conclusion

Do decide to start *today.*
Don't ever stop.